WAR WITHOUT A FRONT
The Memoirs of a French Army Nurse in Vietnam

Elisabeth Sevier with Robert Sevier

WAR WITHOUT A FRONT
The Memoirs of a French Army Nurse in Vietnam

by Elisabeth Sevier
with Robert W. Sevier

Edited by Nancy J. Vesta, M.S.

WESLEY PUBLISHING COMPANY
2704 Blue Quail Pass
Edmond, Oklahoma 73013

©1997 by Elisabeth Sevier
All rights reserved. Published 1999.
Printed in the United States of America

Cover art: French and American Flags by Jennifer Anne Barron, Edmond, OK.
ISBN 0-9652703-1-9

Dedication

War Without A Front *is dedicated to the brave young men and women who served in Vietnam. I would especially like to honor the more than 100,000 French and American patriots who made the supreme sacrifice for their God and country.*

Elisabeth Sevier with Robert Sevier

Table of Contents

Foreword by Dr. Paul Toubas, M.D.	ix
Time Line of Major Events in French Indochina	xiii
Map of Vietnam	xv
Prologue	xvii
Chapter 1—Returning Home	1
Chapter 2—Indochina	11
Chapter 3—Michelle	23
Chapter 4—Tourane	29
Chapter 5—Transfer to Hue	49
Chapter 6—Mouse Trapped	59
Chapter 7—Laos	75
Chapter 8—Rest and Relaxation	81
Chapter 9—Viet Minh Buildup	95
Chapter 10—War Comes Closer	107
Chapter 11—Airborne Training and Return to Laos	115
Chapter 12—Nam Dinh and the End of the Tour	125
Chapter 13—Home at Last	141
Epilogue	145
Endnotes	147
Additional Sources	152
Appendix	153

Elisabeth Sevier with Robert Sevier

Foreword

The story of Elisabeth Sevier covers a major segment of the French Indochina war (1950–53). To understand the motivations of a 20-year-old French woman to participate in the war effort as a nurse, we must recall the extraordinary life of an adolescent girl during the troubled times of French occupation by Germany. Pictures come back to memory, like a black and white movie.

In the Forest of Vincennes, in the afternoon, close to the castle and German Army barracks guarding the eastern part of Paris, a teenage girl, shivering with fright, oscillates on a bicycle. Not too far behind her, also maneuvering on the cobblestones of the road, two armed German soldiers, on similar vehicles, patrolled the surrounding grounds. Elisabeth ignores the nature of the small package she transports on the flimsy carrier of the bicycle. The only recommendation of the man who gave her the package: "Do not be arrested with it." Fearing an imminent confrontation with the German patrol, Elisabeth throws the package in the bushes. Fortunately for her, the slippery wet and unequal cobblestones provides a providential accident. One of the German soldiers falls. A few seconds later, a big explosion rocks the forest. She is now far ahead of the soldiers and understands her luck in avoiding capture.

Soon the clandestine activities of Elisabeth forced her to leave Paris. She had to abandon her mother and younger sister. Her beloved father had died in a German prisoner-of-war camp. She had nothing to lose. The little brunette was transferred to the formal Resistance forces as a *Maquisard* (resistance fighter) of *Reseau Jean Marie*, an organization of the Buckmaster Network (War Office), that specialized in sabotage and parachuting of arms. She met new friends and challenges. Her main participation consisted of carrying messages, capturing parachuted supplies, and caring for wounded partisans. She was only 16 years old and known only as "Lisette." During the next two years, she was constantly confronted by dangerous, unusual, and horrible situations. In 1944, while helping a friend destroy railroad tracks, she was arrested and German soldiers shot the other captured *Maquisards*, including her friend, while she knelt helplessly. The Gestapo and Milice beat and humiliated her. Suddenly, she awoke after a week of questioning and torture to an open and unoccupied jail. The Germans had left because the Allies had retaken the town. She was very weak, fainted, and was taken to a French hospital. Lisette rejoined her Resistance unit and stayed until November 1944 when *Reseau Jean Marie* was incorporated into the First French Army.

As a member of the French Army, Elisabeth served as a nurse and ambulance driver, participating in the Battle of Colmar near the French-German border. Her ambulance was destroyed by artillery fire not far from Colmar and she was injured and her best friend was killed. Only when she returned to Paris and enjoyed a week of freedom and insouciance did Elisabeth have the first really human experience in her young life. However, shortly after her return to duty, she experienced devastating losses of friends and loved ones.

At 18 years, Elisabeth was a veteran of the Resistance and the French Army and was decorated with the French Croix de Guerre for valor during World War II. Elisabeth was discharged on March 16, 1946, and returned to school to get her degree before going on to nursing school. Two years later, with her completed studies, her inextinguishable energy, an innate taste for adventure, independence, and also a sense of mortality, she volunteered for active duty in French Indochina: the first 20th-century Vietnam war, started in 1945. She had knowledge from her high school studies that Indochina was a French colony. She remembered the colorful atlases with all the French territorial possessions. Since 1942, these overseas mysterious countries were not her immediate concern. Her priority had been survival.

The wheels of history continued to turn and the destroying events of the second World War sent different messages across the world. France had been defeated by Germany, and the French Colonial Army in Indochina was mostly destroyed in March 1945 by the Japanese occupying forces' surprise attack, just a few months before the atomic bomb was dropped at Hiroshima.

The Vietnamese people, well educated through the French school system, had developed an acute sense of democratic rules and wanted them to be applied to their people. The prestige of France was gone; it was time to get the keys of the house. Some Vietnamese, like Ho Chi Minh, had developed advanced concepts for the liberation of their people. Rejected and fooled by the French colonialists, he rapidly found sympathy and support from China and the United States, who supported his resistance of the Japanese. The Viet Minh, with Chinese and American help, prevented the weakened French forces from regaining a grip on this large territory. France had not yet understood the futile character of colonial wars and persevered at the reconquest of Indochina. French forces were meager, poorly equipped, but aggressive and composed of young soldiers who had already participated as combat commandos in Europe.

Elisabeth never doubted victory; having fought against the powerful Wehrmacht, the small, thin, Viet Minh rebels did not impress her. The salary was good and when she returned to France, she would have a full degree in nursing. Elisabeth arrived in Saigon on August 20, 1950. Reality quickly sank in. Coming as liberators, the French troops found themselves in the position of occupants. The population was ambivalent. Elisabeth discovered a beautiful country with a difficult climate and the horrors of a new war with an invisible and cruel enemy. She accomplished her duties with the grace and compassion of a young nurse, following troops to the fighting arenas in the jungle. The enemy was not always the Viet Minh. Malaria, typhoid, and amebiasis were common ailments. She suffered through the inescapable vision of torn bodies. She loved, despaired, and left parts of her soul in Vietnam.

Elisabeth Sevier's book is more than a succession of adventures and struggles. For the younger generations, it explains that liberty may be lost and the price to pay for freedom is very high. As other freedom combatants, she paid that price and many of us are alive and free today because of her actions and the actions of countless other courageous people. The book also explains that people have a keen sense of liberty and that our liberty may be servitude to others. Thank you, Madame Sevier, for explaining the meaning of the word—"Liberty."

Dr. Paul Toubas, M.D.
Oklahoma City, Oklahoma

Major Events
French Indochina
October 1950–February 1953

1950

10-08: Viet Minh wipe out French columns at Caobang and That Khe.

10-16: French command abandons 155 kilometers (250 miles) of Chinese border to Viet Minh.

11-20: Viet Minh leaders hold first parley with Laotain and Cambodian rebel chiefs.

12-17: Marshal de Lattre de Tassigny named as High Commissioner and Commander-in-Chief of French Indochina.

1951

1-18: French break Viet Minh attack on Hanoi.

3-15: General de Lattre de Tassigny demands more troops for Vietnam.

4-07: Ho Chi Minh drops formal war against French.

5-31: French troop ship *Adour* explodes in Saigon harbor resulting in 55 dead and 14 injured.

Lieutenant Bernard de Lattre de Tassigny, son of Marshal de Tassigny, killed during actions at Ninh Binh.

9-15: Marshal de Lattre de Tassigny visits United States for purpose of obtaining support for French war in Indochina.

10-03: Viet Minh break French offensive in northeast Vietnam.

11-10: French troops drive Viet Minh from 248 square kilometer (400 square mile) area near Hanoi.

11-14: French paratroopers capture Hoa Binh.

1952

1-11: In Paris, Marshal de Lattre de Tassigny dies of cancer at age 62.

1-15: Guerilla actions by Viet Minh on French troops increase significantly. The son of General LeClerc wounded in battle at Tonkin Delta.

2-24: French evacuate Hoa Binh and regroup for concerted Tonkin Delta drive.

10-05: French troops start first large operation of the year 14 kilometers (22 miles) north of Hanoi along Route 3.

10-29: French begin OPERATION LORRAINE to cut off Viet Minh fuel supply.

11-07: French forces cut off main Viet Minh supply road with China.

11-24: Operations BRETAGNE, ARTOIS, AND NORMANDY launched against 15 Viet Minh battalions near Nam Dinh.

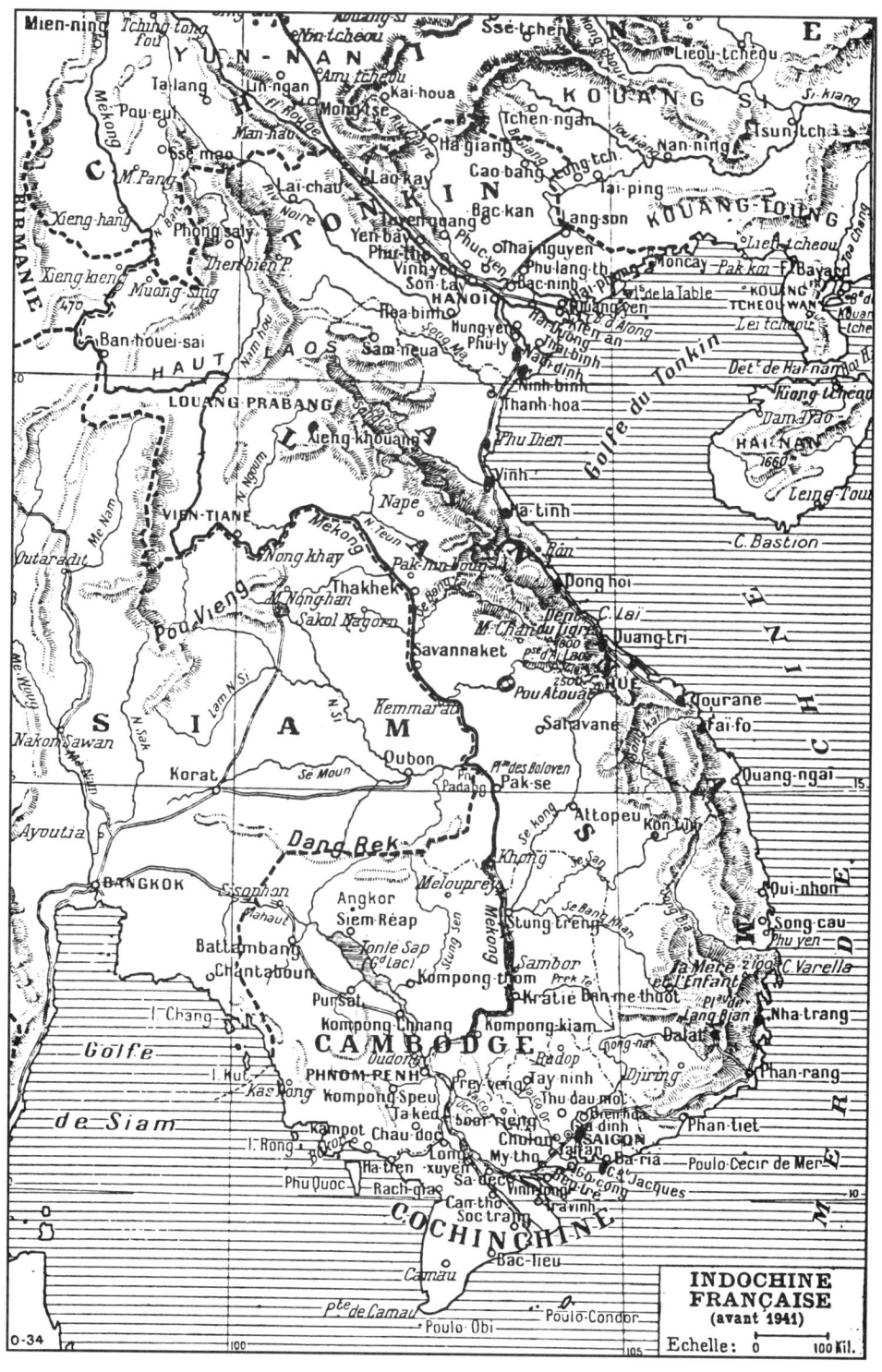

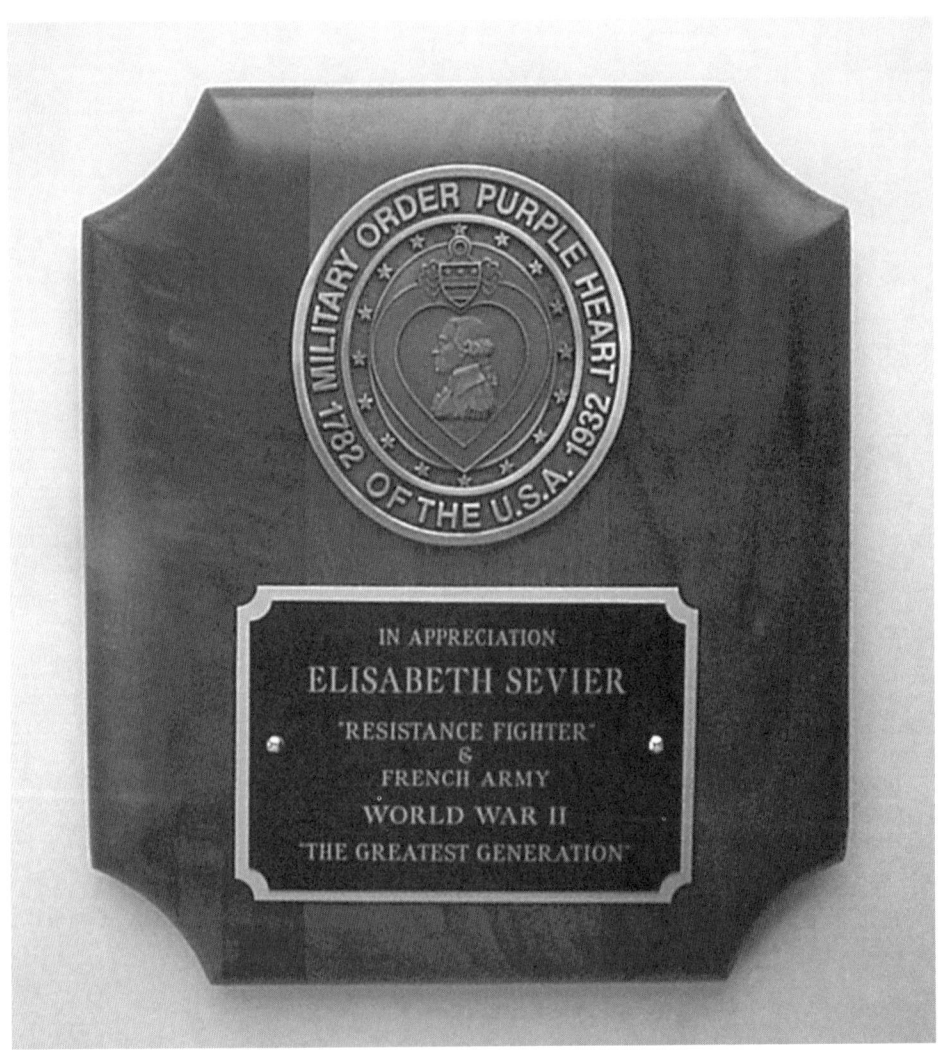

Elisabeth was honored by The National Order of the Purple Heart at their National Convention held in Oklahoma City on August 14, 1999. National Commander Boyd Barclay presented the plaque shown above in appreciation of her services in the French Resistance and the French Army during World War II.

Prologue

War Without A Front is the second book on my life, the first being *Lisette: The Story of a Teen-age Girl in the French Resistance.* The paperback edition of *Lisette* was published as *Resistance Fighter: A Teenage Girl in World War II France.*

At the end of World War II, I was discharged from the French Army and returned to school to become a nurse. After completing school, I decided to go back into the French Army and volunteered for duty in French Indochina.

France captured Saigon in 1859, organized the colony of Cochin China in 1867, and declared protectorates over Tonkin and Annam in 1884. The three were merged with Cambodia in 1887 to form French Indochina. A nationalist movement arose in the early 20th century, gaining momentum during the Japanese occupation in World War II. After the Japanese withdrew in 1945 the Viet Minh, a coalition of nationalists and communists, established a resistance movement headed by Ho Chi Minh. French attempts to control and establish Bao Dai as emperor resulted in the French Indochina War (1946–54), which ended with the French defeat at Dien Bien Phu.

I served in French Indochina from August 17, 1950 to February 25, 1953. My first assignment was in Cap St. Jacques (Vung Tau) which is on the South China Sea south of Saigon. This assignment was regular hospital duty and I soon applied for and received a transfer to Tourane (Da Nang) where I worked as a triage and surgical nurse in medical stations that served French troops in the field.

I was stationed in Tourane then moved to a larger hospital in Hue. In both cases, I spent more than 50 percent of my time as a triage and surgical nurse in the field behind French military lines. The supply of modern medical equipment and medications, especially penicillin, was in extremely short supply during 1950 and 1951; however, we began receiving American help in late 1951 and we had sufficient supplies beginning in early 1952. The French Army also began receiving American equipment including planes and weapons that helped in our operations within Indochina.

The French war in Indochina was fought by regular army, French Foreign Legionnaires, and French Moroccans. No draftees were sent to French Indochina. As time wore on, the French people grew tired of the conflict and the French government essentially abandoned hope of retaining Indochina as a colony. Due to other problems, especially in Algeria and Africa, France did not have the money or the will to win and began looking for a graceful exit from the conflict. However, this was not to be, and the Viet Minh defeated the French in Dien Bien Phu effectively ending French colonization of Indochina.

Dates and names of specific operations and actions of the *Antenne Chirurgical Militaire* (A.C.M.) 507 were verified by the author at the French Army Archives at Chateau de Vincennes in Paris, France.

War Without a Front

Elisabeth Sevier with Robert Sevier

Chapter 1
Returning Home

On March 7, 1946, I was discharged from the French Army and returned to Paris to live at home with Maman, my mother, and Suzanne, my younger sister. My relationship with Maman had always been tenuous and our relationship had further deteriorated when I joined the French Resistance in World War II. Maman did not like the Nazis in Paris, but she worried about my welfare and felt that my boldness would get me killed. However, she welcomed me home after the war, pleased that I had survived past my 18th birthday, and our rapport greatly improved. After moving incognito around the French countryside, administering health care to *Maquisards* (French Resistance members) under primitive conditions, and witnessing the death of most of my friends, I was happy to return to school to finish my baccalaureate (high school degree).

However, in July my knees grew painfully swollen. Maman treated me with home remedies such as applying raw mashed potatoes to my legs. The inflammation receded but the soreness persisted, becoming so great and my fever so high that Maman called Dr. Montan. He immediately arranged for an ambulance to take me to Hospital Tenon. The staff took me to x-ray and then directly to the operating room. When I awoke, my legs were in traction and large needles were inserted in both knees.

The surgeon told me that he had removed a great deal of shrapnel from both knees. I had been wounded when my ambulance was hit by mortar during the Battle at Colmar, but not all the pellets had been removed from my body. After the surgery at Tenon, my knees were still infected; however, the hospital did not have any penicillin. Instead, the doctor reopened both knees and used maggots to cleanse the pus from them. My fever went down slightly, but the doctor told me that if he could not obtain some antibiotic soon, I would lose my legs.

Desperate, I wrote to General Charles De Gaulle explaining my predicament. Since I had been very active in the Resistance, I thought he might take an interest and find a way to help me. I would rather have died than live with amputated legs. Even when I had been captured by the Nazis and faced death, I was not as despondent as when I lay in the Hospital Tenon. Within 24 hours after sending my letter to General De Gaulle, my doctor received the penicillin. In two days, my fever subsided and I began to feel like a human being again.

A week later, General De Gaulle came to see me. His visit was completely unexpected and put the hospital staff into complete ecstasy. General De Gaulle, the leader of the Free French during World War II, was held in the same high esteem in my homeland as Franklin Delano Roosevelt had been in the United States. When I saw him, I almost came unglued: Here was my hero, the savior of my beloved France, bringing flowers for me! He came to my bed, leaned over, and hugged me. He was so tall! I was too overcome to express my gratitude to him and was crying and laughing at the same time. He talked to me a few minutes but I was too excited to process what he said; however, I recall that he had arranged for my continuing care and rehabilitation at an American hospital in Neuilly.

In December 1946, I received an invitation to have tea with General De Gaulle. I took a taxi to his office where I was escorted to a small room and seated. The Louis XIV decor was beautiful—I had never seen such fine furniture. In a few minutes, General De Gaulle came in, shook my hand, and then hugged me. He sat behind a huge mahogany desk and his Aide de Camp poured tea for us. The General had been monitoring my progress and felt happy I was walking again. He asked about my future. I told him that after I completed nurses' training, I planned to rejoin the Army and volunteer for French Indochina. He said, "I wish more citizens were as patriotic as you, Elisabeth." He congratulated me for my decision, wished me his best, and then departed. His administrative assistant came into the room, asked me a few questions about my life, home, and family. He thanked me for coming and escorted me outside to the street where I took a taxi back home.

Despite my injuries, I was walking on air: I felt tremendously honored to have been received on invitation to talk with General De Gaulle. I will always be grateful for his personal intervention to obtain penicillin and arrange for my treatment. Later, he also assisted in acquiring my citizenship. I had been born on a boat in the Mediterranean, as my mother fled from an Armenian concentration camp after World War I, and was officially a Greek citizen. With General De Gaulle's help, I became a French citizen on May 11, 1947.

In June of 1948, I completed my baccalaureate with the assistance of tutors provided by the French government for homebound students. (Even with therapy, I could not walk for three months after leaving Neuilly and I continued treatments for 18 months on an outpatient basis until my wounds entirely healed.) I was a good student and was pleased to receive my diploma, but I had a greater honor bestowed on me at that time. On June 10, I was awarded the Croix de Guerre with bronze cross for my service in the Resistance. The ceremony was held at the Invalides in Paris where approximately 30 *Maquisards* were honored for their valor during World War II. Many of the decorations were given posthumously. As the survivors received awards for the heroic deeds performed by persons I had known and loved, I cried for the survivors, the dead, and myself.

I began nursing school in October 1948 with morning classes at the Sorbonne and practical training in the afternoons at Salpetriere Hospital in Paris. The 16 months of school and time with my family were happy days. However, I had never been a particularly patient person and after being a nurse in World War II, I found routine hospital duties boring. Consequently, I was anxious to finish school and complete my training in the Army where I could work in the field. I was especially fond of and proficient in triage, a relatively new process of handling casualties where the soldiers were brought to a central area and the seriousness of their wounds evaluated. Those with injuries requiring immediate attention were treated in the field while those with less serious wounds were stabilized and transported to nearby hospitals for treatment.

I informed Maman about my decision and as I thought, she was unhappy. She had expected me to complete training and remain with her in Paris. She was upset, but I was now of legal age and she could do little about my choices.

I reenlisted in the French Army on March 24, 1950. I was assigned to Dr. Larrey at the Military Hospital in Versailles where one side of the Palace of Versailles was used for the veterans' hospital. I looked down the rows and rows of patients, wondering if prior to World War II anyone could have imagined the Palace as a hospital for our sick and wounded soldiers. Amidst the splendid rich gold tones, dark woods, and ornate ceilings with crystal chandeliers, the Spartan cots of the patients looked out of place. At the Palace, we received wounded veterans from French Indochina and I familiarized myself with the illnesses common in Southeast Asia. I had never worked with patients who had tropical diseases and it appeared that all our veterans were sick with malaria or dysentery. Most of the men were between 18 and 25 years of age; many were paralyzed or suffered with missing limbs, broken bones, and horrible flesh wounds. Their conditions made me sad, but I never let them know how I felt. I always showed them a smiling face and offered cheerful conversation. I only cried when I was alone. Every day I prayed I could help their morale and give them hope.

I treated three young men for whom I had great concern. Each was in critical condition, very near death. Every time I checked on them their statuses were deteriorating. Their minds and bodies were so enfeebled by the shock of battle and impaired by physical wounds that regardless of the constant attention given to them, they rapidly lost strength. I continually appealed to God to spare them. One night when I was coming on duty, I found one of the other nurses clearly distraught. She told me how she had tried so hard to save a young patient, "I did my best, but it was not enough." Within the next few hours, all three of my patients died also.

During my service in the Resistance, some of my patients had died of injuries or from lack of the will to live. As I gained more experience, I avoided getting emotionally close to my patients, but I never really adjusted to the losses. And some men, especially those who were young, I grieved over a great deal, as if all the tragedies I had seen were manifested in them. This time was no different; I went off by myself and cried and cried. In the morgue, I said my last good-bye to the three soldiers from Indochina. They lay there peacefully, so very young and innocent. I said a prayer for all three of them and left.

I was not always successful in keeping my distance from a patient. One day while working in the Palace, I met a young man named Roger, who was extremely ill with malaria. His fever ranged between 104 and 105 degrees. I administered nivaquine shots and quinine tablets to help, but his was an intense case and he responded slowly to the medication. I changed his sheets almost every hour for five days because of his heavy perspiration. He was also recovering from wounds in his chest and stomach. Finally, after almost a week, he began to recover. He was feeling better and I stopped by and joked with him each day so he would not give way to despair and loneliness. We became fast friends and I felt I was helping him to overcome his extreme depression. He told me that he had been in love with a German girl named Paula. She had left him for someone else, and he had volunteered for French Indochina to forget her. He had almost completed his 24-month tour overseas when he was wounded. My heart sank when he was discharged, but he promised to write often.

I received two letters from him and in the second one, he wrote that he loved me and wanted to marry me. I was flabbergasted. Roger had talked so much about Paula, I knew he still had deep feelings for her. I decided to meet him at his Auxerre home to talk about our futures. I took a one-week furlough and we spent several days together talking seriously. He was a first lieutenant in artillery and wanted to make the military his career and I was already committed to French Indochina. He promised that after his six-month convalescence leave, he would follow me to Vietnam.

I had developed strong feelings for him. He was a handsome man, about six feet tall, with blonde hair and blue eyes. I found him fascinating and felt sorry for him. He was depressed and wounded and had experiences that I understood. I had been engaged to an American pilot who died in the final weeks of World War II and could relate to his feelings of loss over Paula. I also struggled with depression. I had lost my father and my youth to the cruelest of wars. I had grown up in Catholic boarding schools and felt very little warmth from my own mother. Consequently, my fellow *Maquisards* had become my family and most of them were dead. My best friend had married and moved to America. I was only 20 years old and very much alone. Therefore, though I was afraid he was marrying me on the rebound, he assuaged my feelings, and I, eager for someone to love me and to feel some sense of belonging, accepted his proposal.

We were married on August 3, 1950, with ceremonies both in a Protestant church in Paris and city hall. Maman was upset because I was not married in the Catholic church, the first in my family to marry outside the faith, and none of my relatives attended the wedding. Our honeymoon lasted only two days because I had to report back to the hospital. We spent the time, which was exceptionally happy, in Auxerre at Roger's parents' home.

Elisabeth Sevier with Robert Sevier

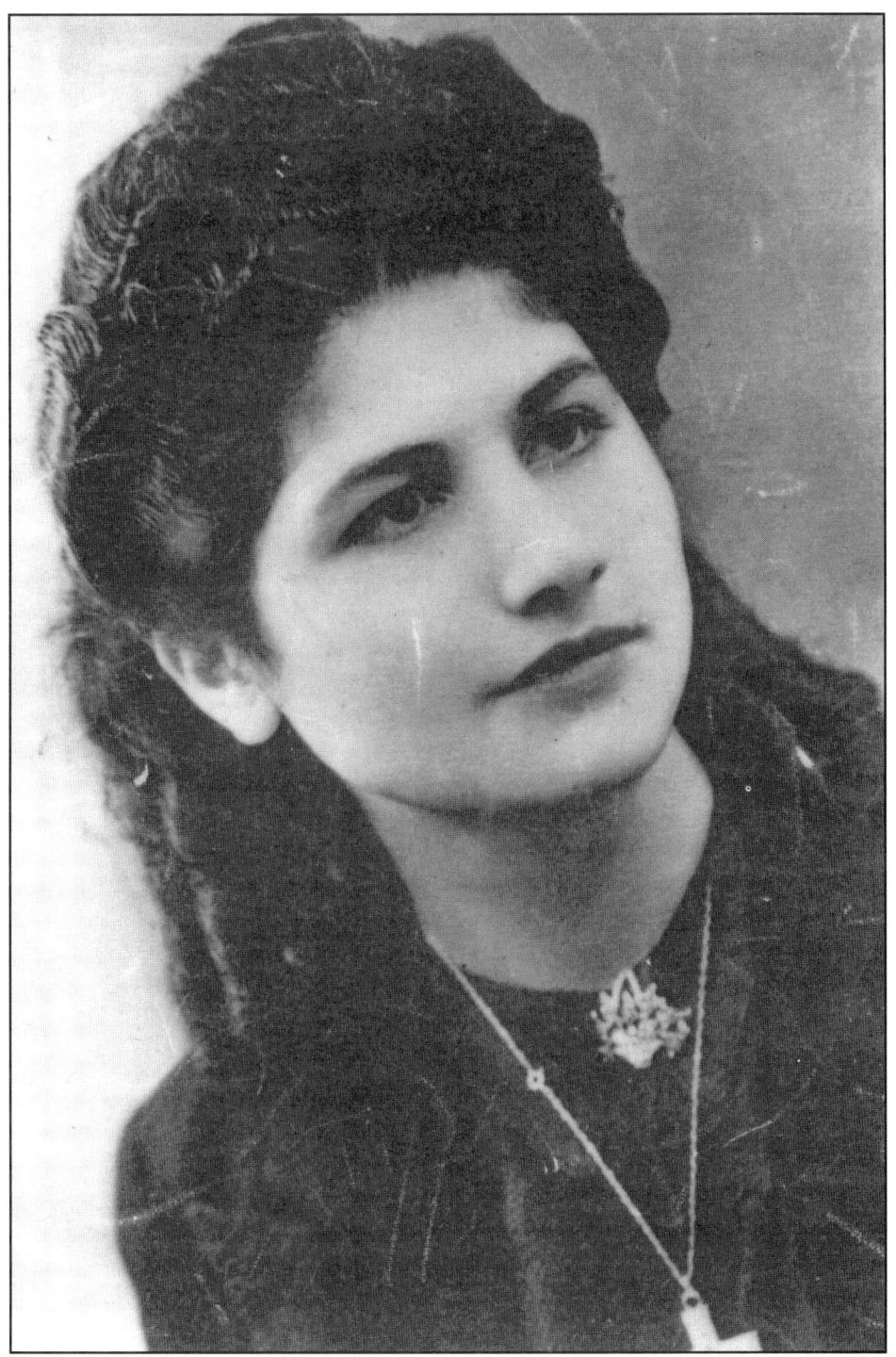
Elisabeth — age 20

Elisabeth Sevier with Robert Sevier

Chapter 2
Indochina

On August 17, 1950, I left Paris on a military plane and landed in Saigon three days later. Roger had seen me off at the airport and promised he would follow me within a month. I felt terrible about leaving Roger so soon, before we had time to really get to know each other. I also realized that I had married too soon. I loved him very much but I intuitively knew that he did not reciprocate the same intense feelings I had for him. Therefore, my heart was heavy at my departure.

On the plane to French Indochina I met Margaret, also a nurse, and we quickly became friends. Margaret was a beautiful girl, taller than I was, with brown hair and brown eyes. She was 25 years old. After we arrived, Margaret and I took a tac-a-tac (pedicab) all over Saigon taking in the sights and sounds. The city smelled horrible, because of the polluted Saigon River, and was unbearably hot, about 95 degrees, and extremely humid.

The next day, we went shopping. The captain had told us to always travel with someone and never be alone in the city.[1] We went to a French cafe, then to a French movie which had Vietnamese subtitles, and to a Vietnamese restaurant. Afterward, we hailed a pedicab and asked the driver to take us to a place where we could get drinks and have fun. He took us to an old building crowded with young people, including quite a few soldiers, but most patrons were French and native civilians who worked for the French government.

We could not find a table inside and ended up on the outdoor patio where six old men smoking long pipes sat in a circle on the floor. They were very animated and seemed happy. They asked us to join them. We were hesitant, but we did not have anywhere else to sit. They extended a pipe to each of us. Wishing to be polite, we tried to smoke, imitating them. Just one puff caused both of us to begin uncontrollable coughing. The old men just sat back and laughed. We felt very sheepish and kept on smoking to show them that we were worldly adults. After a few puffs, we did not remember anything. We woke up on the patio floor at six o'clock the next morning feeling horrible, as if we had been drunk for a week. We were sick to our stomachs and had violent headaches. When we stood up, both of us immediately threw up all over the floor. The manager gave us some coffee and advised us to never use opium again. We were both aghast; we had not even considered the fact that the men might have been smoking dope. The bartender said, "Most Indochinese men have used opium all their life but French women are just too delicate to handle it." Contrite, we went back to the hospital by pedicab.

The next morning, Margaret and I traveled three hours by boat to Cap St. Jacques, located 100 kilometers from Saigon on the South China Sea. Against a backdrop of breathtaking mountains, the extraordinary foliage made Cap St. Jacques beautiful. However, I was to learn that many Viet Minh (communists led by Ho Chi Minh) were using the lush mountain vegetation to ambush the French and native allies into brief engagements that almost always put the French on the defensive and hurt morale. We were assigned to the service of Dr. Lariat, Colonel and Director of the hospital. He received us graciously and I immediately felt welcome.

Margaret and I were taken to a small, 10-room hotel where we would be living. The front double door was guarded by the

Mamadou, black soldiers from the French Congo, who ensured that nonresidents, even guests, did not enter our hotel. They were exceptionally polite but never looked directly at us or spoke casually with us.

Margaret and I were amazed at the number and diversity of the insects and rodents we saw since our arrival in Indochina. The rats were huge; some looked like mid-sized cats. We had to be extremely careful not to leave any food on the floors, tables, or countertops and we always slept with mosquito netting firmly in place to protect ourselves from disease-carrying mosquitoes and other insects. We also welcomed the small white lizards, who made a home on our ceilings where they ate insects and were considered good luck charms by the Vietnamese.

We reported to the U-shaped, 200-bed hospital the day after we moved into our apartments. Two nurses were assigned to each wing and I was lucky enough to be working with Margaret.

After three days on duty, I was asked to give a strychnine shot to a Mamadou patient who had dysentery. I went to his bed, pulled back the sheets, and was startled as he immediately began to scream in a language I could not understand. I turned and began to walk away, but he got up from the bed and began to follow me, screaming and gesturing in a threatening way. When I got to the end of the hall, all the doctors and nurses were laughing as I ran for my life. Dr. Lariat calmed the patient and then told me, "I asked you to treat him to teach you a valuable lesson." He continued by telling me that the Mamadous did not believe that women were capable of treating them and the native men were afraid of them. Consequently, 20 French Foreign Legion male paramedics cared for the wounded blacks. Only when the Mamadous were under anesthesia were they touched by women nurses.

At night, the Viet Minh infiltrated Cap St. Jacques and destroyed supplies. Most of our soldiers lived in the city and patrolled the surrounding countryside during the nights. Their primary mission was to protect the large rubber plantations which were owned by the French. When they were wounded in action, we flew them to the large Saigon military hospital. When the planes could not hold them all, they were evacuated by boat. However, boat travel was dangerous for our medics and wounded soldiers. The Viet Minh used hollow bamboo stalks to breathe while they swam underwater to plant explosives on the boats.

Margaret and I both loved the beach and spent many hours taking in the sun and watching the boats. One day while swimming, we saw a smoking plane approaching extremely fast. It crashed into the mountains and we were horrified. We had recognized the medical transport plane, suffering from obvious mechanical malfunction, and realized that one of our friends, a nurse named Renee, was on board. She was burned beyond recognition and for the first time since arriving in Vietnam, I felt vulnerable.

I settled into the routine of working in the hospital and spent most of my off-duty hours writing home and visiting with Margaret and Monique, a beautiful girl from Martinique. She was 10 years older than I was and a perceptive person. As our friendship grew, she asked why I was so sad.

I had been in Indochina for more than four months and had not received even one letter from Roger. I had religiously written to him—at least three times each week—but never received a reply from him. I also discovered that I was pregnant. Feeling abandoned by my husband and afraid that my superiors would send me back to France if my pregnancy was discovered, my sadness degenerated into depression.

The progress of the war in Indochina did not help my disposition. Shortly before I arrived in September 1950, the Viet Minh launched their first major offensives in the northern territories. In their usual hit-and-retreat manner, they attacked poorly manned French outposts. When the French pulled the plug on the forts and the inhabitants, which often included civilian support staff and their families, retreated, they were often ambushed in the thick jungle. In addition, valuable supplies, in which the Viet Minh were in desperate need, were left behind.[2] The Chinese, who had capitulated to the communists, could now send supplies to the Viet Minh, unhindered, down northern Indochinese trails.

After losing a major offensive in the rice paddies of southern Vietnam in 1950,[3] the Viet Minh never engaged the French in an up-front battle. They always attacked and retreated, leaving rubble and death, but no enemy to fight. Consequently, French casualties and frustration mounted.[4] The French were never able to use their superior resources in the isolated, small, jungle trails. Stories from the north, the monsoon rains, and the constant raids in the countryside deflated morale.

In late 1950, we received some uplifting news: General de Lattre de Tassigny had been appointed the High Commissioner and Commander-in-Chief for French Indochina. I was especially happy because I had served under him in the First French Army during World War II. When General de Lattre de Tassigny arrived in Saigon on December 17, 1950, morale improved throughout Indochina because we felt he would lead us to victory.

Elisabeth Sevier with Robert Sevier

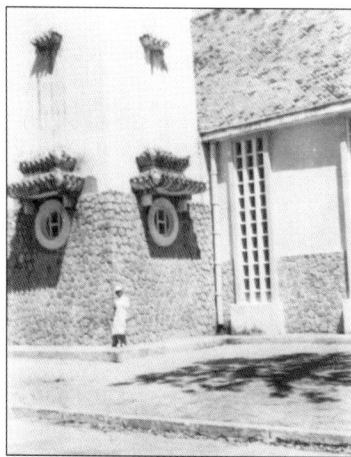

French headquarters — Saigon

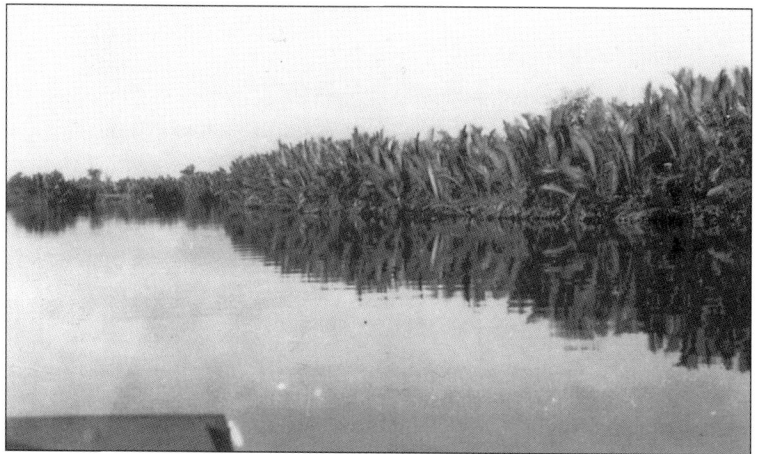

Boat trip from Saigon to Cap St. Jacques

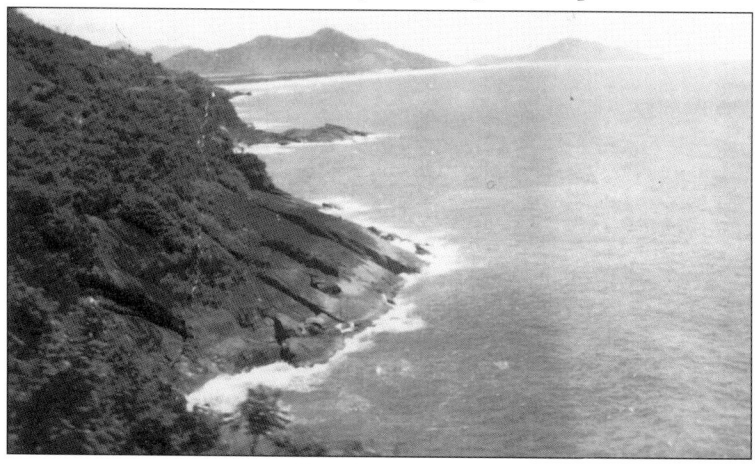

Cap St. Jacques

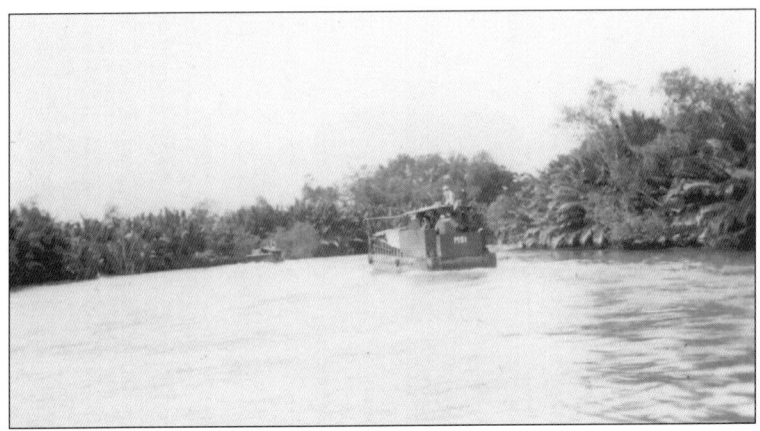

Boat trip from Saigon to Cap St. Jacques

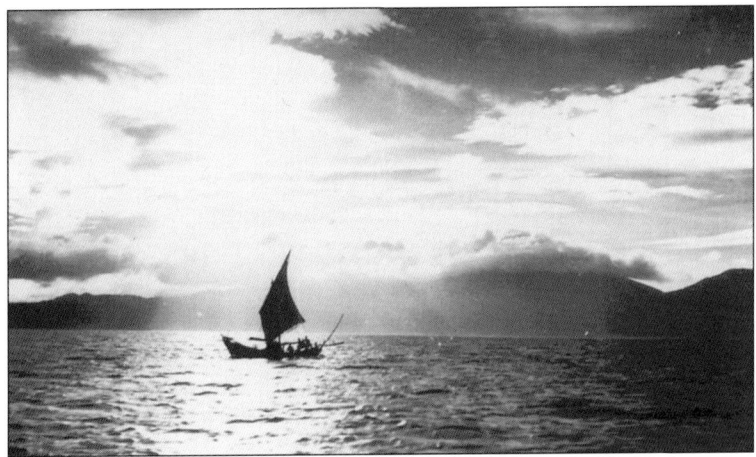

South China Sea at Cap St. Jacques

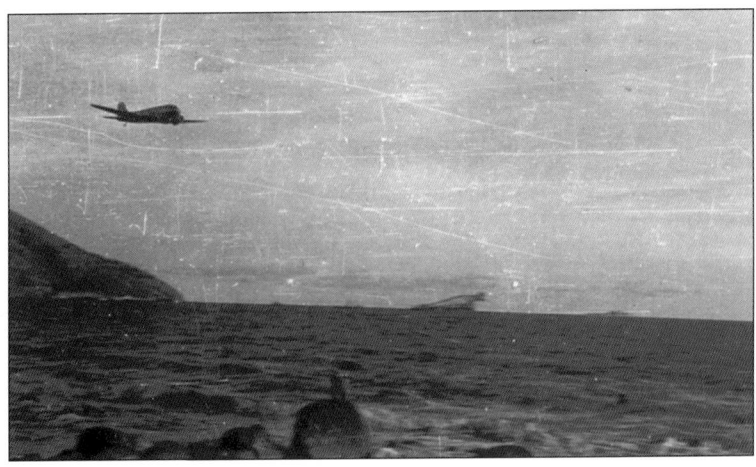

Cap St. Jacques

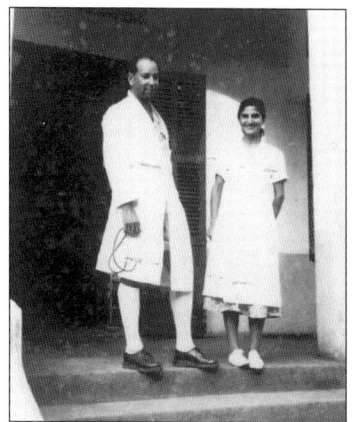
Dr. Lariat — Elisabeth

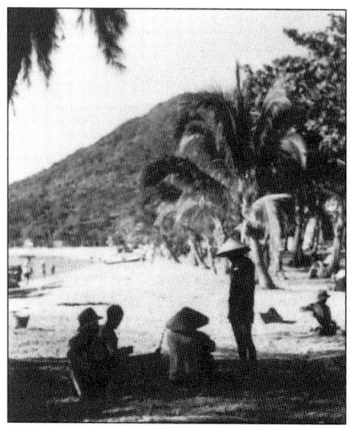
Beach at Cap St. Jacques

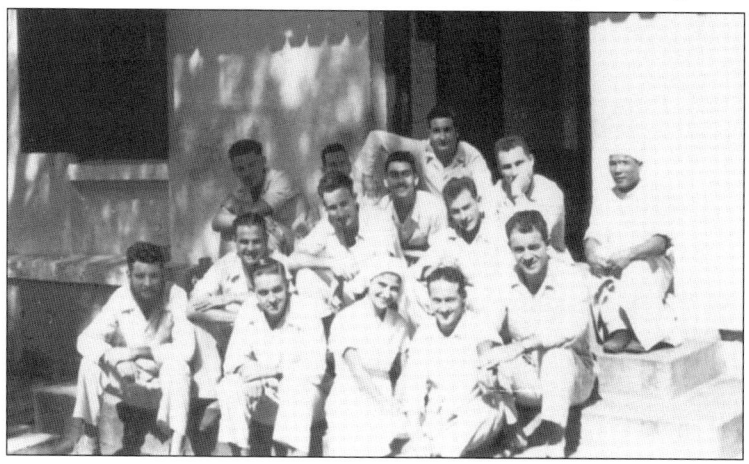
Paramedics at Cap St. Jacques

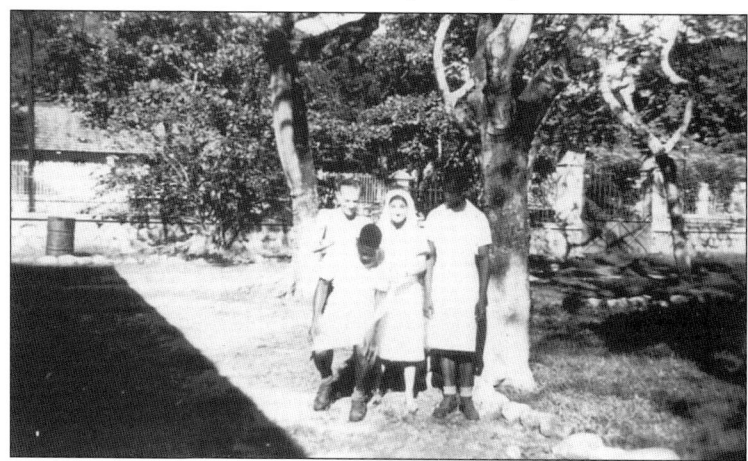
Elisabeth with Mamadou guards

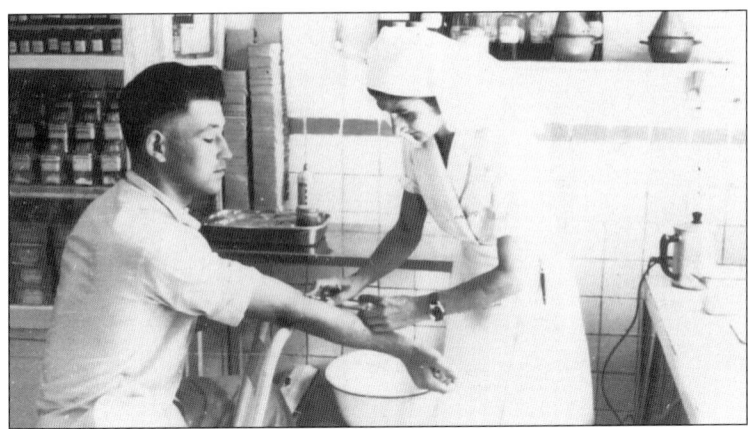
Treating a patient

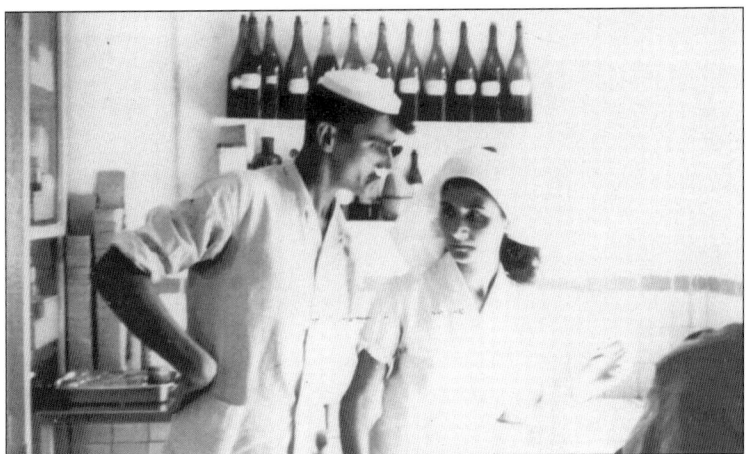
Elisabeth and paramedic

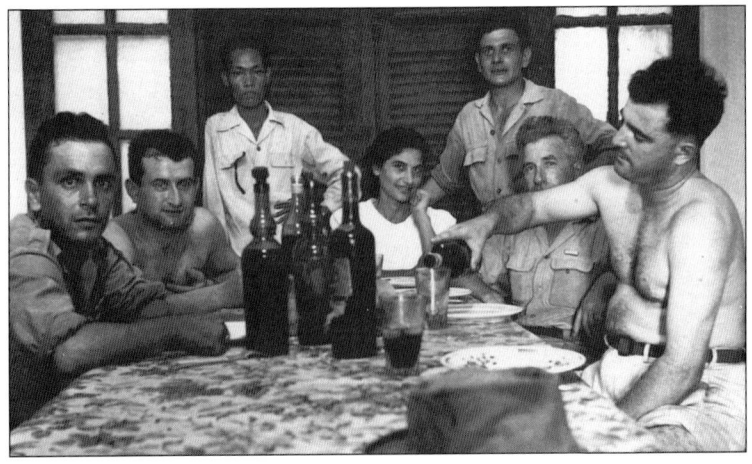
Elisabeth with legionnaire paramedics in Cap St. Jacques

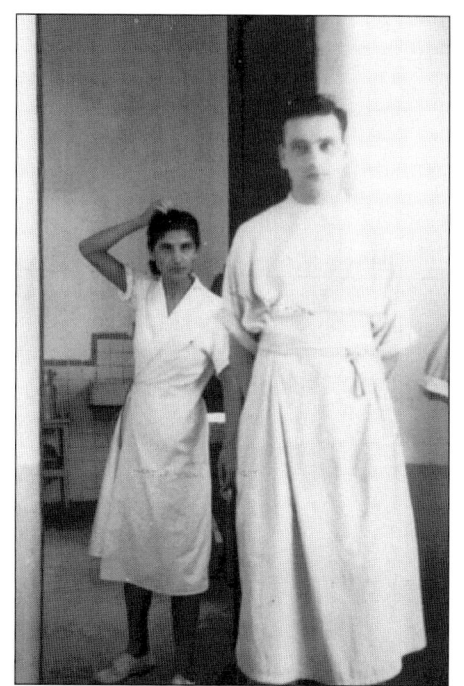
Elisabeth and paramedic

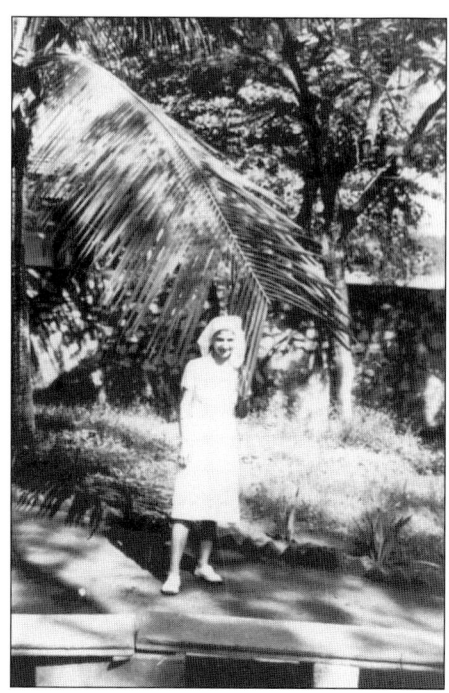
Elisabeth

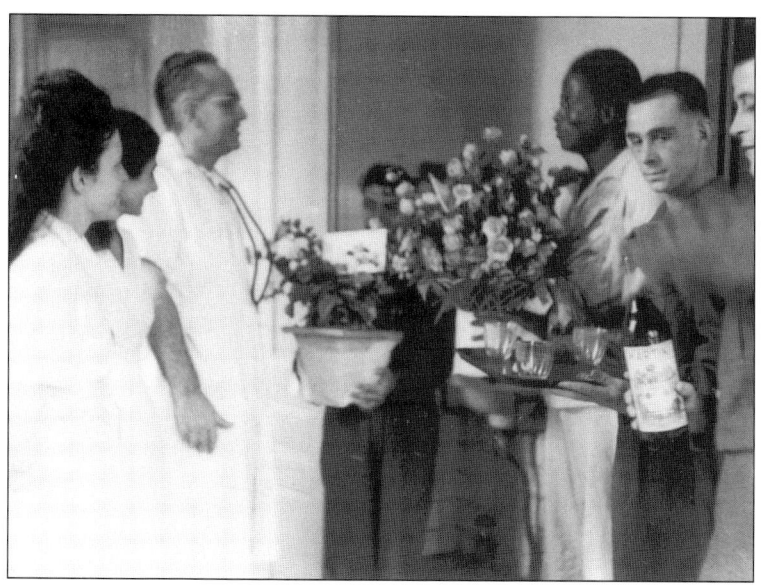
Christmas at Cap St. Jacques

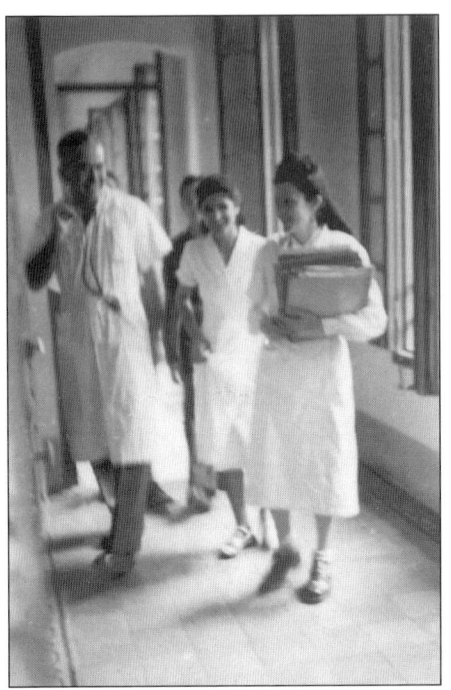

Dr. Carpentier, Elisabeth, and Lilliane

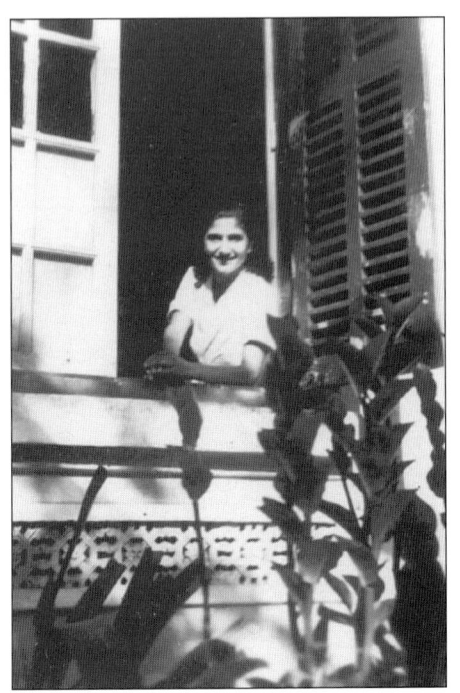

Elisabeth at hospital

Chapter 3
Michelle

*I*t was the Christmas season and Margaret, Monique, and I celebrated together. We arranged lights in the form of a tree in each hospital ward. We sat together with most of our patients in a circle holding hands and singing Christmas carols. As we sang "Sainte Nuit" ("Holy Night"), my eyes were filled with tears as I remembered holidays of my past. Before World War II, Christmas was a happy time for me and my extended family. We always had a beautiful tree, wonderful dinners, presents, and songs. However, after the Nazis occupied Paris, I spent most holidays at boarding school. When I was home, my family's losses weighed heavily on Maman, Suzanne, and I. We endured food rationing, lack of heat for our apartment, and ice-cold bath water. My father was captured and died in a prison camp, my sister, Annick, died of tuberculosis, and my aunt and cousins were killed by Luftwaffe strafing while they fled to the countryside in a refugee convoy.

Christmas in 1950 was most like that of 1944, when I had spent the day with wounded soldiers in a freezing Colmar Pocket hospital ward, singing the same carols and feeling the same sadness about my past. However, in Indochina, I also longed for Roger and wondered why I had not received any letters from him. I pulled myself from depression by recognizing that Roger's feelings were out of my control. Though I could not do anything about my marriage, I concentrated on having a healthy baby.

In my eighth month of pregnancy, I could no longer hide it and I told the doctors and staff that I was going to deliver a baby soon. They supported me in every way. I hired a maid who helped with normal household duties; however, I was able to continue work until May 24, 1951, when after a difficult labor and delivery, I gave birth to a beautiful baby girl. She had blue eyes like her father and a head full of light brown hair. She weighed four pounds, three ounces, and required 24-hour hospital care for the first month of her life. I named her Michelle in memory of my best friend and fellow *Maquisard* who had been killed during the Battle of Colmar. I was ecstatic when I was able to take her from the hospital. I hired a native nurse to take care of Michelle when I was working, but I could hardly wait for each duty day to end so I could return home to my baby.

Michelle was thriving until one day early in July. I received a call from my nurse who said that Michelle was very ill. My baby was immediately admitted to the hospital with acute dysentery and within three days she was dead. We buried her tiny body in a small French military cemetery that overlooked the sea in Cap St. Jacques. I had never told Roger or my family that I was pregnant, hoping to surprise them with the happy news. When Michelle died, I was alone again, devastated, and in shock: I could not believe that I had lost my little girl. My friends at the hospital helped me through those desperate days.

It is ironic that shortly after Michelle died, I received the first letter from my husband. He was coming to Cap St. Jacques and needed to talk to me. Disillusioned and suffering, I did not want to see him. What could he say to me that would alleviate my pain and loneliness? How could he possibly make up for abandoning me and our baby? I volunteered for duty as a field nurse in central Vietnam so I would not have to see him. I signed on for an additional two years in Indochina to get the transfer and I was delighted that Margaret decided to join me. Though we were issued orders right away, they did not come fast enough. The evening before we were to leave, Roger came to the beach where we were swimming. "Please stay so we can work out our problems," he begged.

"No," I said directly. I told him the sorrow, torment, and depression his broken promises and lack of communication had caused me.

"I didn't come here or write because I visited Paula in Germany. I'm still in love with her . . . I love you both and must sort this out."

I was not surprised or bothered by his confession. However, his complete disregard about his own daughter astonished me. He did not care at all about her or what her suffering and death had done to me. I was disgusted with him and any love I had left for him disappeared. However, I was raised Catholic and divorce went against my ingrained beliefs. "I will never forgive you, but I will not give you a divorce while I'm in Indochina."

"I will follow you where ever you go until I get a divorce," he said angrily.

Elisabeth Sevier with Robert Sevier

War Without a Front

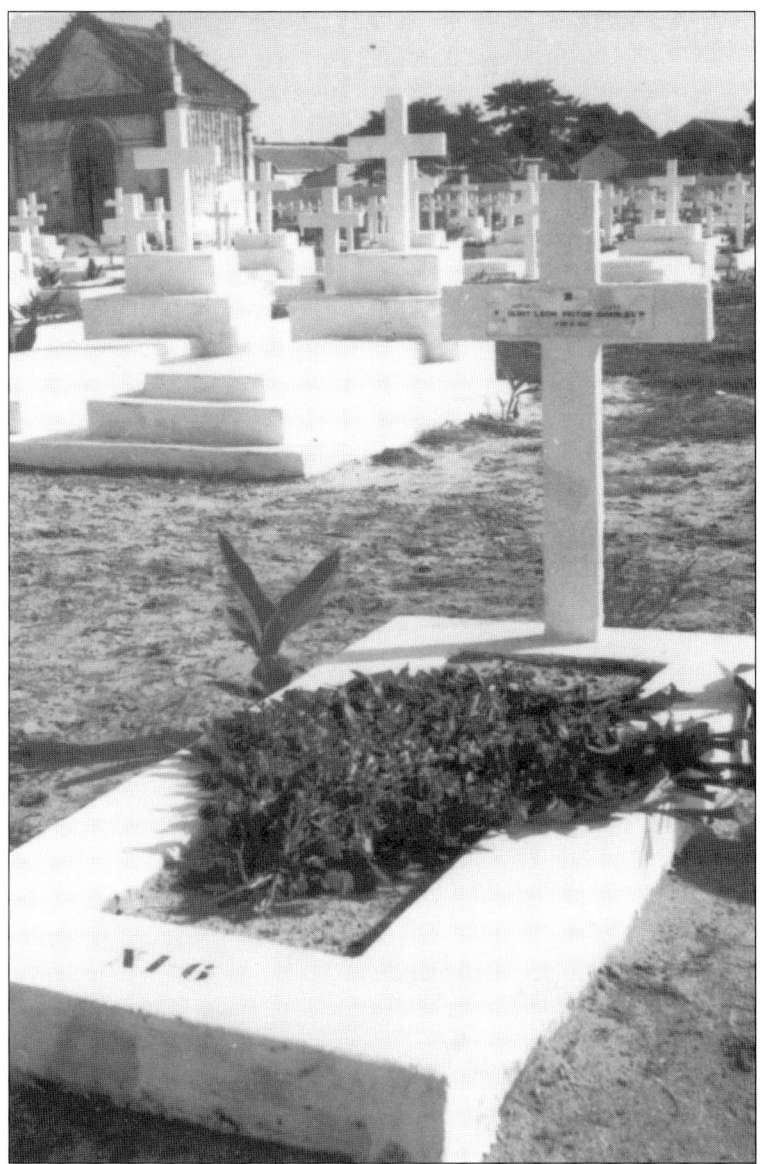

French cemetary at Cap St. Jacques

Elisabeth Sevier with Robert Sevier

Chapter 4
Tourane

The next day I left by convey with Margaret for Tourane (now called Da Nang) to *Antenne Chirurgical Militaire* (ACM) 507 to serve as a field nurse. Tourane was a fairly secure garrison, but Margaret and I were assigned with 2 other nurses, 2 doctors, and 12 French Foreign Legion Paramedics to set up surgical stations in areas of intense fighting. Our triage units were the precursors to the American Army Mobile Surgical Hospitals (M.A.S.H.), first used extensively during the Korean War. Tourane reached 95 degrees with 100 percent humidity so we were required to wear cotton uniforms. Nylon would burn our skin in the intense heat.

We did not go into the field right away but settled into a small, but comfortable, hotel. We worked in a 50-patient ward, tending troops brought in from the jungle. Each of the nurses had a small office where she sat and completed patients' charts. All the treatments performed and all medications given were noted. Paramedics returned the completed records to the patients' beds. On subsequent rounds, nurses would check to ensure that all charts had been returned to the proper patient. Four nurses split the duty cycle in the garrison hospital. We worked in eight-hour shifts with one nurse available for the operating room. The morning shift started at seven o'clock and terminated at three o'clock.

The afternoon shift only consisted of one nurse and two paramedics as did the third shift which began at 11 o'clock at night. We used 30 minutes of each shift to brief our relief nurse on the progress and status of each patient. I volunteered for night duty because the quieter atmosphere gave me time to talk to the soldiers and listen to their comments, problems, and concerns. During the night, I made rounds every half-hour to ensure that the men were as comfortable as possible.

Doctors, nurses, and paramedics ate in the hospital at mess-hall tables which would seat 25 people. The legionnaires were in charge of the mess facility and the cook was a legionnaire. The food was very good, although plain, consisting mostly of fish, chicken, duck, and beef. We also enjoyed fresh vegetables from local markets (although these had to be disinfected in a bleach solution). We also had plenty of red table wine from France.

Frequently, we went to downtown Tourane where excellent restaurants served Vietnamese dishes. I especially loved the spring rolls with chicken, and the soups were particularly delicious. Most of the Vietnamese people, especially the educated, spoke fluent French and it was easy to communicate. Overall, the Vietnamese people were very nice to us; Vietnam had been a French colony since 1888 and most of the middle-class civilians made careers in French government and industry.

I was only in Tourane for a month when Roger showed up for his divorce. "I made a mistake in marrying you. I really love Paula."

I knew that Roger and I could never live together as man and wife, but I felt strongly that divorce was against God's will. An annulment was acceptable, but I could not obtain one when away from France. To compound my anxiety over the separation, I was confused about how the marriage had gone awry. I prayed for a solution and by the end of the summer, I realized that divorce was, indeed, the only solution. I felt the burden being lifted from my soul as I prepared the legal papers.

While I was feeling better about my future, I was treating patients who faced many uncertainties about their own lives. Though the fighting had subsided in our area, we routinely handled dysentary, which we treated with emetine and strychnine, and malaria for which we used quinine; however, many men died before responding to treatment.

Even when combat was slow, not all cases were routine. One night, just after finishing my third round, the paramedics brought a young Vietnamese soldier from the French Army into the emergency room. His color was ashen and his breathing labored. I administered a saline-solution IV (intravenously administered medication) to replenish his fluids and called Dr. Carpentier immediately. He arrived within five minutes and stated that the young man had amebic dysentery. He was put on emetine, but did not respond; he suffered profuse diarrhea and intense bleeding. We gave him strychnine shots to help his breathing, but I had to change his sheets every hour. When I changed his bedding for the third time, I saw not only blood, but also two-inch, flat, white worms in his discharge. His stomach had extended to balloon-like dimensions and was extremely taut. I immediately called the doctor who informed me the worms were commonly called "suckers" and usually were fatal.[5] We administered plasma, but had no penicillin so we gave him sulfa to fight the infection. I called Margaret and she helped with the other patients while I attended the young Vietnamese. He was in such pain that I had to administer morphine in large doses to ease his agony. He died early the next morning. His was the worst case of a parasitic infection I had ever seen and it was shocking. I prayed that I would never contract suckers. I went home but could not sleep and had nightmares about the case for months afterward.

One morning a blaring bugle woke me up. I did not realize that we were under enemy attack but the garrison immediately prepared for action. We packed up our medical supplies, tent, instruments, and cots and loaded them into trucks. We were told that the enemy was near Quang Tri (Vung Tau), approximately 150 kilometers north of Tourane, near the 17th parallel that would later divide Vietnam into North and South.

Our medical detachment consisted of one doctor, Dr. David Carpentier, and three nurses—Margaret, Danielle, and me. Travel was slow because the roads were rough and dotted with mines. We arrived at a point near Quang Tri and carefully chose the sight for our medical unit. We had to select an area protected by trees but near a flat spot or level road where a small airplane could land and evacuate our badly wounded patients. We had two small aircraft that could transport two patients at a time. We set up our operating-room tent, a patient tent which held about 20 soldiers, and tents for the nurses and paramedics. The surgery tent was large enough to accommodate three separate operating areas and Dr. Carpentier decided to sleep there. We had been joined by 12 Foreign Legion paramedics who had helped us set up facilities. Within an hour after we established our unit, casualties began to arrive.

We sorted out the incoming patients and established priorities for treatment. As soon as we had stabilized them, the more wounded patients were immediately airlifted to the main military hospitals in Tourane and Hue. The less seriously injured were transported by ambulance to Quang Tri and then put on the train to Tourane or Hue. We worked for two days around the clock with no respite. News spread that French troops had been ambushed outside Quang Tri and most were massacred. We treated more than 100 patients within the week. Dr. Carpentier had to call another physician, Dr. Lariat, from Hue to help him. We also welcomed another much-needed nurse, Monica. In many cases, the nurses assisted in surgery and closed the patient's wounds so the doctors could move onto other critically injured soldiers. I had never seen so many casualties at one time. After the wounded had been treated and moved, we attended a mass funeral in Quang Tri for the 220 French soldiers who had been killed during the ambush.

We cleaned the operating-room tent and I was overwhelmed with the copious amounts of blood everywhere. With the help of the paramedics and Vietnamese of the French Colonial Forces, we disinfected the supplies and packed the tents within a week. We placed the instruments in open-weave wicker baskets so air could circulate through them and mildew would not form.

The medical equipment issued to us was outdated and often inadequate. We were still using red rubber tubing for catheters and operating procedures because plastic tubing was not available. Some instruments were so old I did not recognize their purpose and we only had one 1930s-vintage autoclave to sterilize them. Although we had plenty of morphine and blood plasma (we never used whole blood which could carry malaria and other diseases), we were always short of penicillin. Consequently, we used sulfa drugs extensively to treat infections.

The soldiers also suffered with obsolete World War II equipment discarded by the American Army. Most of their small arms were M-1 rifles. The soldiers also had American tanks and mobile artillery, which were difficult to maintain in combat-serviceable condition in such high heat and humidity. Large equipment was also difficult to use on small jungle passes. The French made more use of two and one-half ton American trucks, but they had difficulty obtaining parts for repairs.

Morale was horrible. Despite General de Lattre de Tassigny's best efforts to drum up support in the homeland, France was obligated to post-war European stability and could only commit North African troops as reinforcements.[6] His campaign was better received in the West where Mao Tse-tung's Chinese revolution created concern about the spread of communism. In 1950, America, notorious for its anti-colonial sentiments, dispassionately provided funding and equipment to keep the French forces viable enough to prevent a complete communist takeover.[7]

However, only regular French Army troops and mercenaries[8] were sent to the area, so no real public support was generated among the war-weary French population; the war, increasingly funded by the United States, did not affect them.[9] In fact, some French, including paratroopers sent in 1945 to liberate Indochina from the Viet Minh, were hostile toward the colonists who they perceived as Japanese collaborators. Though right after World War II Allied forces had been able to recapture areas like Saigon from the Viet Minh, the French had been ineffective at eliminating the nationalist leader, Ho Chi Minh.[10]

Upon seeing the suffering of our soldiers, I, too, wondered why we were fighting in Indochina. I remembered how I despised the Germans when they occupied Paris. So, I understood the Vietnamese quest for independence and their motives to fight against French colonialism. However, when I could think clearly, put the images of shattered bodies out of my mind, I realized communism was not going to free the Vietnamese. I felt we could and should save long-time Vietnamese loyalists of France from a repressive and cruel dictator such as Ho Chi Minh.

So, though my work was not as clear-cut as when France was fighting Hitler, I reminded myself that innocent people were still endangered by a revolution that would mean misery to those under conquest. Therefore, when in November 1951 we received 200 new medical recruits from France, I gladly helped them join our efforts. We carefully checked their immunization records and set up briefings about the hazards of living in central Vietnam. We warned them not to swim in the rivers, told them to disinfect rural drinking water, and suggested that when in cities or towns they only consume bottled water or wine. We taught them how to detect dysentery, malaria, and typhoid. We emphasized the need to use mosquito netting whenever resting or sleeping.

I also took advantage of the chance to help the civilian population when Dr. Lariat needed volunteers for the annual French medical visit to the leprosarium near Da Lat. Margaret, Danielle, and I went with him to set up an aid station. The self-contained village housed 90 people, all of whom had leprosy. While in the leprosarium, the patients could roam freely, but if they left the compound they had to wear bells around their necks to signify that they were lepers. Because leprosy is such a contagious disease, most of the Vietnamese treatment colonies were in or near the mountains away from the general population. I had never treated leprosy before—none of our wounded soldiers had been afflicted—and I wore rubber gloves for protection. We stayed for two days and treated many women and children for minor problems, but most of the men refused to be seen.

In early December 1951, we were again deployed near Quang Tri where Dr. Lariat, Margaret, and I set up our medical site nearby. The soldiers told us they had been on patrol and while crossing a swampy area, had been ambushed by snipers in nearby trees. They never saw their enemy. Only two or three soldiers had been fortunate enough to escape without injury. About one-half of the patrol of 35 men were new recruits—boys who had been in the country less than a month. The most seriously wounded were evacuated by small aircraft, and those without life-threatening injuries were transported to Tourane by ambulance. We quickly ran out of medicine and bandages and had to order a resupply which came by air.

I was riding in an ambulance, using plasma and sulfa to treat a young man with leg wounds, when despair overcame me. The futility of what was now a political war and the images of cruelty, accumulated through years of working in backwoods field hospitals in Europe and Asia, distracted me and for the first time in all my war-time experiences, I wanted to go home. My homesickness was intensified because I had recently received a letter from my sister, Suzanne, telling me that she missed me and that she hoped I would be home for Christmas. When I focused again on my patient, I shook my head and resolved to stop feeling sorry for myself. I thanked God that I was not in the condition he was in.

We arrived at the Tourane hospital where I immediately put on my scrubs and began helping in the operating room with Dr. Lariat and Margaret. We had only ether and chloroform for anesthesia, both of which caused pain and nausea after its administration, but we were lucky because we had just enough penicillin for the eight patients who needed surgery. We worked throughout the night, completing the last operation at eight o'clock the next morning. We had a quick breakfast with coffee and then went to the lounge where we slept on cots the rest of the day and night. The legionnaire paramedics manned the hospital nursing duties while we slept. If a patient became critical, all the doctors and nurses were available to help.

Because I felt safe, I was in good spirits upon returning to Tourane and settled into routine hospital work. After completing rounds, Dr. Carpentier gave us instructions for each patient. Margaret took one side of the ward and I tended the other. We also had two paramedics each to help us. They changed the bedding, washed the patients, and helped feed those who could not eat by themselves. In general, the paramedics attended to the less sick while the nurses concentrated on the more critically ill patients, who had curtains drawn around their beds to signify that only the nurses and doctors were to attend to them. We were all extremely careful to ensure that mosquito netting was tucked in completely to protect the patients.

Overall, we were grossly understaffed, especially during times of crisis when we had many casualties from operations near the area. Dr. Carpentier taught us the duties of a circulating nurse and a scrub specialist. We had two operating rooms which were connected together at the hospital. Although not a surgeon, Dr.

Lariat frequently stepped in and handled the more routine operations during critical times.

Despite the oppressive heat, the intense pain we witnessed, the torrents of blood, and the endless frustration of a misunderstood (and often misdirected) war, we found happiness in our friendships. For Dr. Carpentier and Danielle, their relationship blossomed into love. They were wed in a civil ceremony in Tourane and in a Catholic service on the base. We wished them well on their brief Da Lat honeymoon. Even though my own marital state still caused me great anxiety, I was hopeful for the deserving young couple and wished them years of happiness.

I was ready for some fun too. Since the winter monsoon season was in full swing, military action slowed somewhat.[11] So, Margaret and I took leave to celebrate my 21st birthday. We left on December 14 for Hue in a motor-pool jeep, driven by a young Vietnamese whose family lived in Hue. The roads were rough, but the scenery was dazzling, complete with majestic mountains and rolling valleys. As we traveled, we saw people working alongside their water buffalo in the rice paddies. We checked into our beautiful hotel at Hue. It was managed by a Frenchman who graciously did not charge us for the room or our food when he learned it was my birthday. We enjoyed a large room with a private bathroom and a balcony overlooking the garden.

After resting for about an hour, we went downstairs for a lunch of onion soup, which we had not enjoyed for a long time, and chicken. It was delicious, as was the glass of French white wine. The owner joined us and shared his opinion that the French presence in Indochina was almost over. He had a Vietnamese wife and two beautiful children, and though he was convinced that the French Army would leave, he said, "I will remain in Vietnam regardless of the outcome." After lunch, he prepared an itinerary for us and we happily began our tour.

We took a pedicab to the Then Mu Pagoda located on the left bank of the Perfume River. It was a magnificent structure; the seven tiers of the octagonal tower each represented a different reincarnation of Buddha. As we entered the temple, we had to take off our shoes. The temple boasted an enormous bell—more than 4,000 pounds—which was cast in 1701. The spectacular gardens kept us enchanted the rest of the day.

We woke up early the next morning and after eating, took a pedicab to the Imperial Palace and spent the rest of the morning sightseeing. We had lunch downtown at a Vietnamese restaurant where we ordered spring rolls, chicken Lorraine, white wine, and fortune cookies for dessert. The meal was delicious and the service was excellent. Shopping was next on our agenda and each of us bought a Vietnamese costume, pants with colorful blouses that reached just below our knees. We intended to use the latter as nightgowns.

We returned to the hotel at seven o'clock in the evening and listened to a Vietnamese musical group playing in the lounge. They sang both French and Vietnamese songs. When they sang the French songs, we felt homesick and talked about when we would return home. Margaret had only six more months before going home to Verdun. "Two years is enough," she said when I asked if she would extend her tour. She planned to work at the American base near her family's home. Margaret and I admired the Americans very much. They had rescued France from a life under the Nazis and every American I had ever met, including those downed airmen I treated when in the French Resistance, was cordial and spirited.

The hotel owner invited us to the bar where he toasted my birthday. He then told the bartender to give us a dozen oysters each. Neither of us had eaten oysters on the half-shell before. He told us to squirt lemon on them, put the shell to our mouth, and swallow the oyster whole. They were very good and I ordered another plate but Margaret was not up to it. The owner also had a birthday dinner prepared for me: a thin Vietnamese soup flavored with an extremely hot anchovy-extract sauce; filet of shark served with onion, lemon, and parsley; and small, baked, new potatoes. The meal ended with a French dessert of napoleons and brandy. After drinking cafe au lait (coffee with milk), we thanked our host and walked around the hotel garden before retiring for the rest of our enjoyable evening.

At three o'clock in the morning, I woke up very sick to my stomach. As I rose to go to the bathroom, I vomited. I fell to the floor and crawled to the commode where I continued throwing up. I also had diarrhea and was bleeding. I woke Margaret, but she was also sick and too weak to get out of bed. Eventually, she was able to call the manager who summoned an ambulance for us. We managed to make it inside the vehicle with the help of the medics. They took us to the military hospital emergency room. I was unconscious and remained so for two days. When I awoke, I saw Margaret in the bed next to mine. Panicked, I said, "We'll be absent without leave if we don't report in!" Margaret laughed and told me that I was in the hospital and everything had been taken care of. We were both diagnosed with acute dysentery, so we remained in the hospital for several days.

The last day we were in the hospital, I thought I saw an angel. A lady dressed in white had donned a veil similar to those worn by French nurses. There was a man with her. They stayed all afternoon and prayed for us. We learned that they were American Christian missionaries, Paul and Ruth Carlson from Minnesota. They had been in Vietnam for more than 10 years. The next morning, they brought us flowers and oranges to take back to Tourane and invited us to visit their home next time we came to Hue.

When we were released, the doctor told us that the oysters had made us sick; we should not eat them in Vietnam. When the ambulance arrived to take us back to Tourane, the entire staff lined up and wished us well. Dr. Carpentier gave us another three days off to recuperate and regain our strength. I was happy to be back with my unit, and I hoped I would never finish another birthday celebration in a hospital bed.

I still felt very weak when I returned to work, but Christmas was approaching and we tried to get into a festive mood. The holidays were generally not a happy time for the staff because we were so far away from our families. However, our patients, often critically ill with painful wounds and debilitating diseases, needed as much support and holiday cheer as possible.

I could not help feeling sorry for myself, especially when I began thinking about Roger. I had filed the divorce papers with the French courts, but they had not yet been finalized. I also had the distinct premonition that Roger was coming and I really did not want to see him. I tried not to think about it, but I just could not remove the sadness from my mind. I felt responsible because our marriage had not worked out and guilty about the divorce.

Work must go on though, so I proceeded with rounds and did my best to make the patients laugh and feel good about themselves. The mail came and we received three newspapers from France which were eagerly passed along to all the staff and patients. Mail was a welcome surprise because our postal service was quite unreliable. We often went two weeks without receiving any correspondence. I did not receive any letters from Maman or Suzanne and wondered what was going on at home.

On Christmas Eve the hospital was decorated as attractively as possible. We had cut a small tree and decorated it with candles and fruit. Our patients had also made decorations to put on the tree and we held a small gathering of the entire staff, the patients, and the chaplain, who prayed for all of us and then led the singing of traditional French Christmas songs. It was not much, but it made us come together. We felt a part of something because of our common experiences: We were all a long way from home, fighting a war of attrition that was not appreciated by either the Vietnamese or the French.

The Red Cross came to the hospital on Christmas day and brought small gifts, including chocolate, candy, fruit, and cigarettes, for all our patients and staff. They also distributed personal items such as new toothbrushes, toothpaste, and shaving supplies.

I was depressed on Christmas day because I had not received mail from home and I felt alone. I was tired of the heat, filth, and poor living conditions so I spoke to Margaret and persuaded her to transfer with me to the larger hospital in Hue. We would have modern equipment and more personnel; we had been on duty most of the time in Tourane because we were so short staffed. Dr. Carpentier said he must have replacements before he could even consider the transfer.

To make the staffing situation even worse, three legionnaires deserted within a week. The French Foreign Legionnaires were excellent medics and well trained. However, many were also alcoholics. Some had prior criminal records and volunteered for service in Indochina so that after their five-year tour of duty ended, their records would be expunged. Many legionnaire paramedics married or cohabitated with Vietnamese women and deserted the French Army, which had neither the time nor resources to track them down.

After Christmas, life returned to normal. Duty at the hospital became routine and we slowly began to dissipate our patient load. The monsoon-induced slowdown did not decrease the number of patients with malaria and dysentery.

One day, I went to my office and noticed that a photograph of my sister had disappeared. A legionnaire paramedic had recently tried to befriend me. He was 30 years old, handsome with blue eyes, and could be charming. However, I did not like or trust him. He was a known liar and braggart. He always talked about my sister, how pretty she was, and how he was going to meet and marry her when he returned to France. I knew immediately that he had stolen Suzanne's picture from my desk because he had asked me numerous times for a photograph of her. Unfortunately, Suzanne had written her name and address on the back of the picture.

I told Dr. Carpentier of my suspicions and requested that he speak with the legionnaire about returning my picture. I then talked to some of the other paramedics. They said that he had been showing the picture around, telling them that I had given it to him because he was in love with Suzanne and was going to marry her. They thought it very strange because they knew he had never met or talked with my sister. After Dr. Carpentier talked to him, my photograph was returned when I was away from the office.

We learned General de Lattre de Tassigny had left Vietnam because of illness and was hospitalized in Neuilly in December 1951. On January 11, 1952, we received the news that he had died. It was a sad day for all of us. The General had been a true hero of France and he had managed to give hope and some victories to the troops in Indochina. He was replaced by another highly decorated World War II veteran, General Raoul Salan.

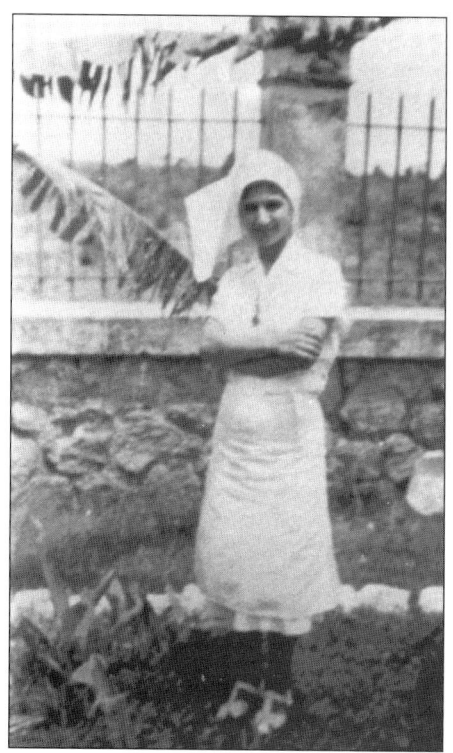
Elisabeth at hospital grounds — Tourane

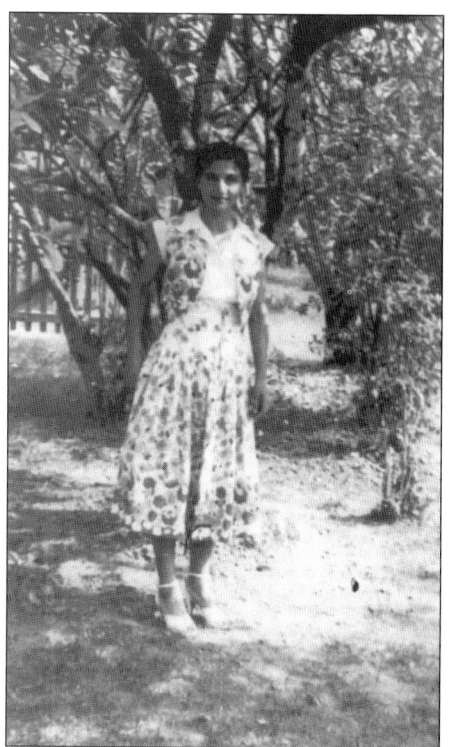
Elisabeth at home in Tourane

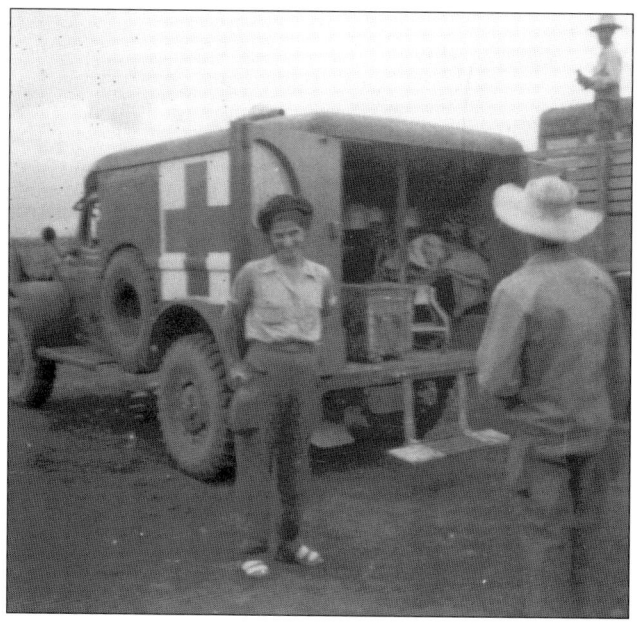
Wicker basket in back of ambulance

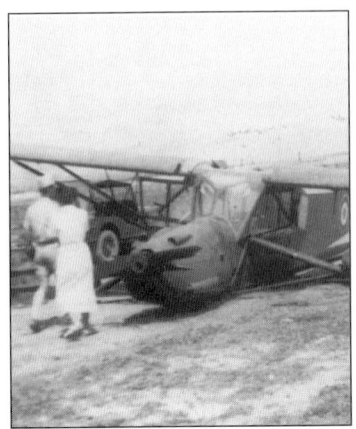
Disabled aircraft near Quang Tri

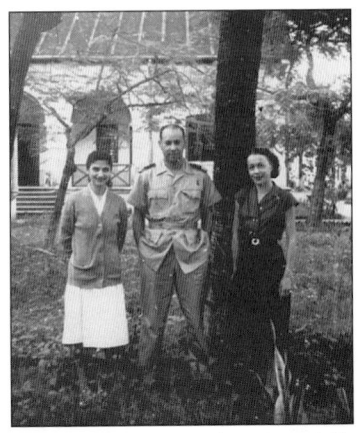
Elisabeth, Dr. Lariat, Danielle

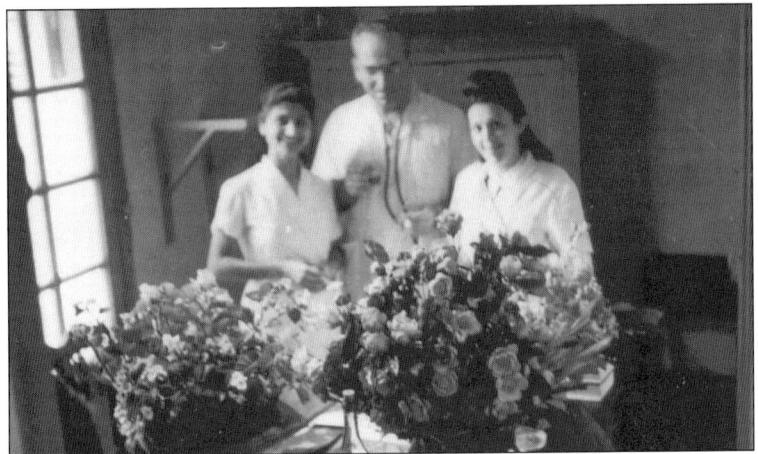
Elisabeth, Dr. Carpentier, Lilliane

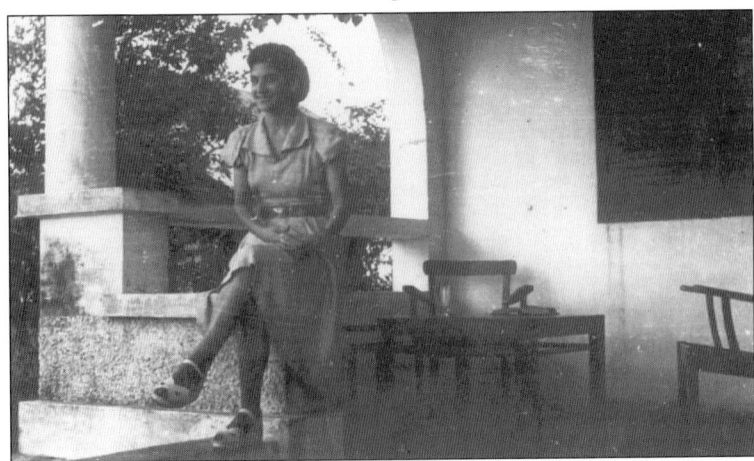
House in Tourane

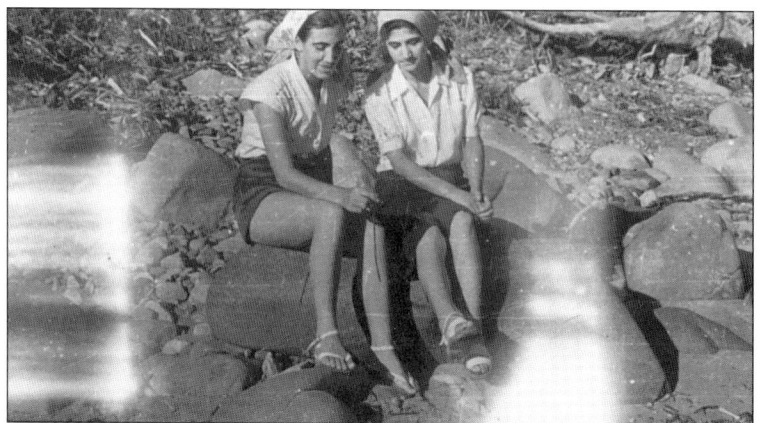
Margaret and Elisabeth

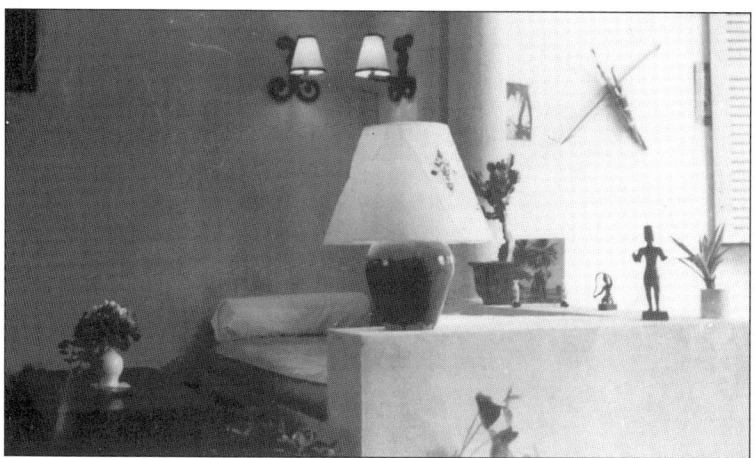
Elisabeth's bedroom in Tourane

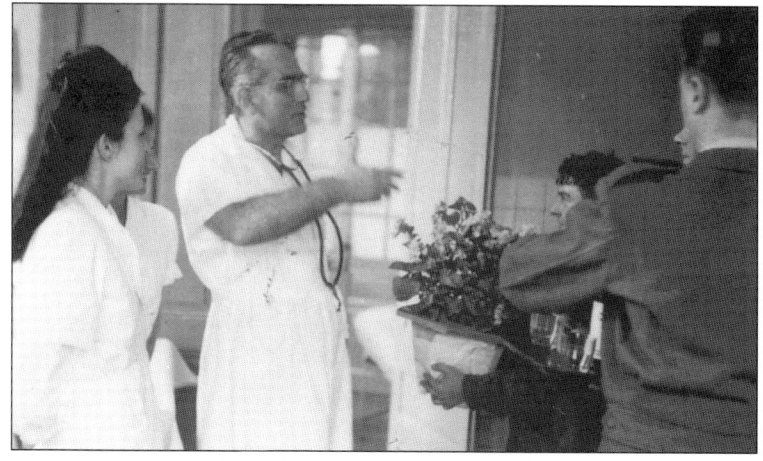
Elisabeth — Dr. Carpentier

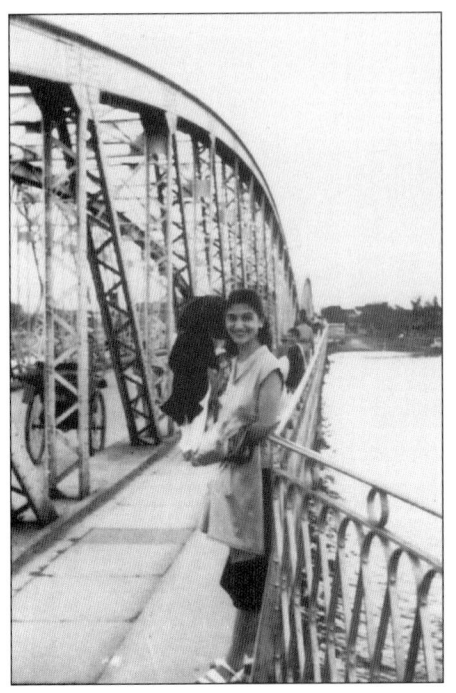
Elisabeth

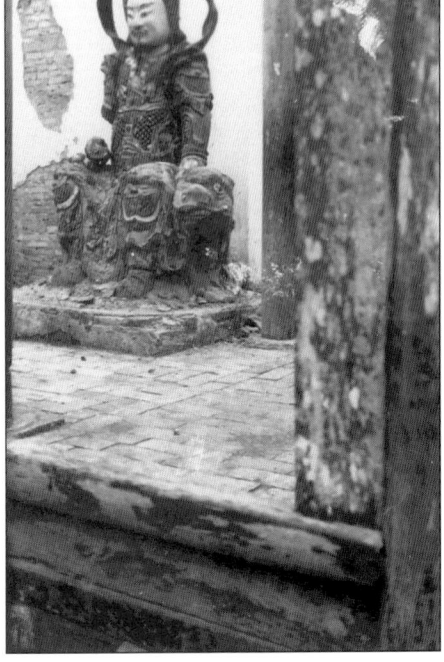
Museum in Tourane

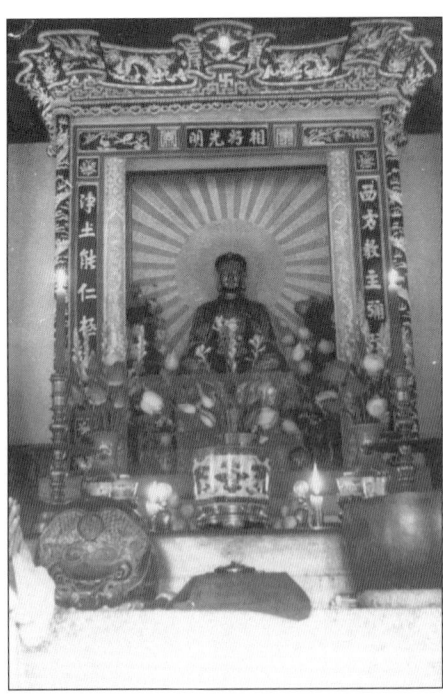
Museum in Tourane

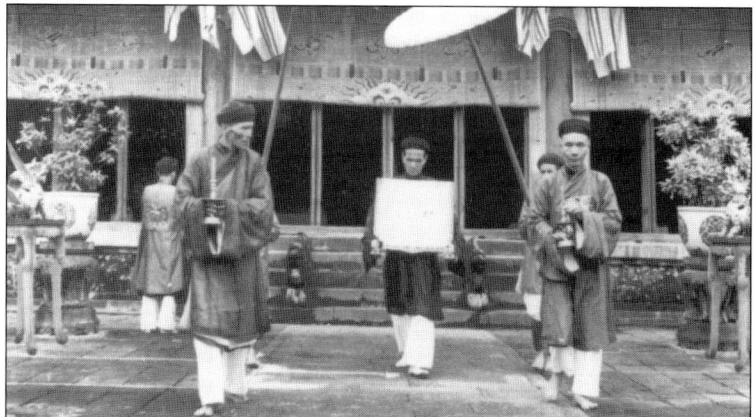
Museum in Tourane

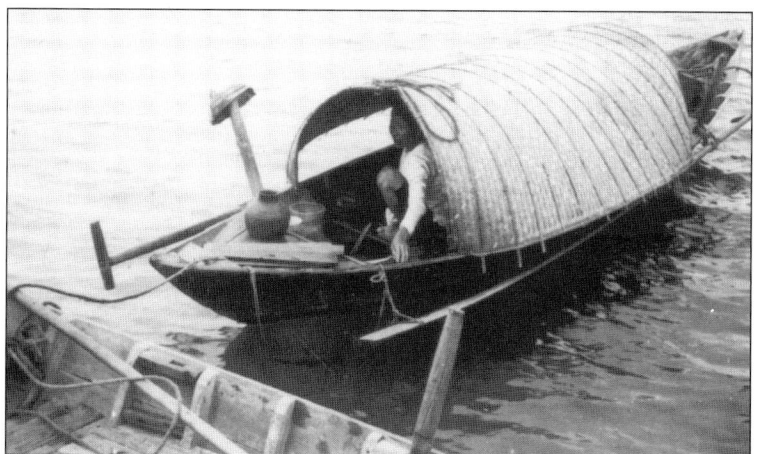
Sampan

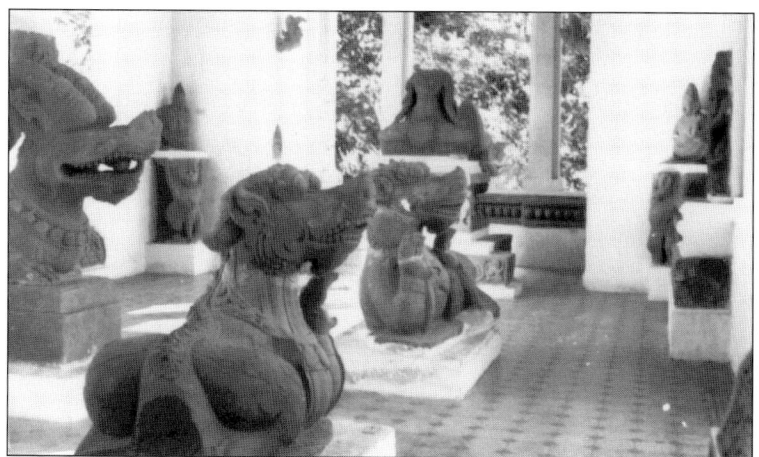
Museum in Tourane

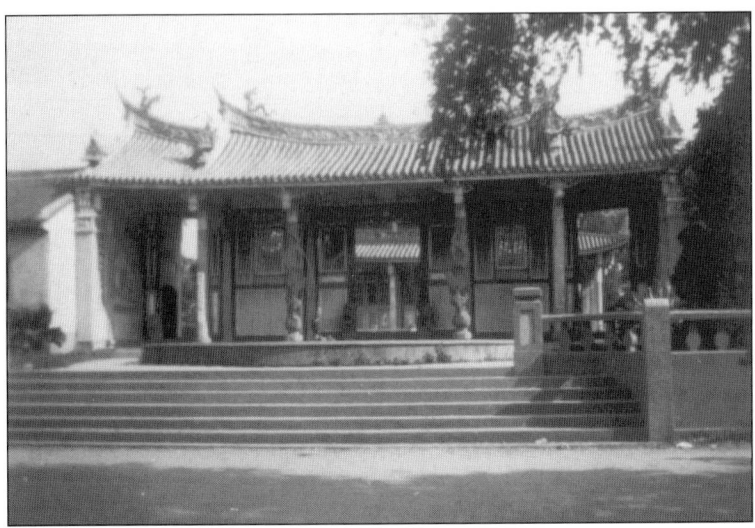

Museum in Tourane

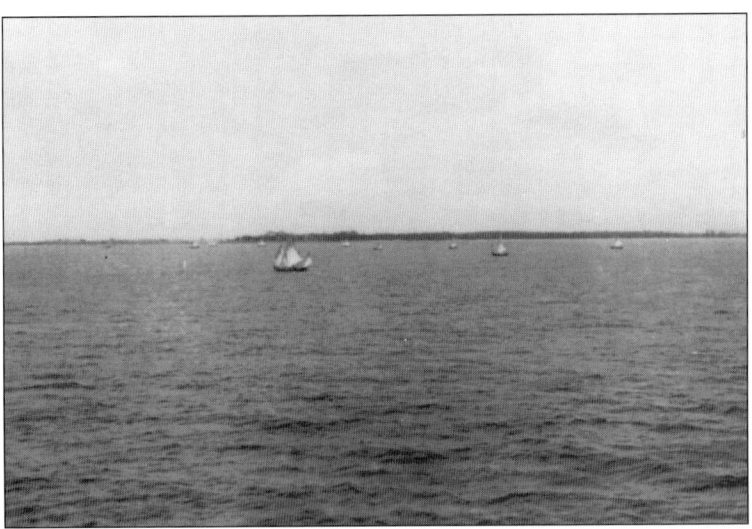

Tourane (Da Nang)

Chapter 5
Transfer to Hue

In early January, Margaret and I were notified that our transfer to Hue had been approved. Dr. Carpentier, who was scheduled to leave in two weeks, had arranged for our replacements. Margaret and I were sure he had personally found the two nurses so we could transfer to Hue before he left. He told us that we would be working much harder in Hue because the French were soon going to expand operations in central Vietnam. He also thanked us for our service at Tourane and invited us to a party that evening.

We met at a small cafe in Tourane and the entire staff, including Dr. Carpentier, Danielle, Dr. Lariat, and Monica, was there to send us off. We had a French meal prepared by the mess sergeant of the Tourane garrison. Margaret and I were almost in tears when the party ended. It was always difficult to leave good friends.

Margaret and I woke up early the next morning and met our driver and armed guard at seven o'clock. We arrived at the hospital in Hue about noon and were assigned to the service of Dr. Deit, the Chief of Staff. Our new quarters were in a small house within walking distance of the hospital. A maid and a cook prepared our meals and kept house for us. We were both amazed at the luxurious arrangement. We each had our own bedroom and shared a bath. The house included a living room, dining room, kitchen, and a front porch with chairs.

With 100 beds, the Hue hospital was much larger than the one in Tourane. It had three operating rooms, an intensive care unit, five ambulances, and was well equipped. With the exception of the large military hospital (Cholon) in Saigon, it was the most modern in Vietnam.

Dr. Deit, a Parisian, was a 35-years-old surgeon who had been in Indochina for six months. He told us that he had received excellent references about us from Drs. Carpentier and Lariat. We also met Dr. Seuzier, who was also a young surgeon. The staff included 7 nurses, 3 legionnaire paramedics, and 20 Vietnamese paramedics assigned to the hospital. Most of the personnel were new to the hospital in Hue, but had served at other facilities in Vietnam. Consequently, all the nurses were familiar with triage, were knowledgeable in the treatment of colonial diseases, and were cross trained as operating room nurses. The Vietnamese paramedics were also excellently trained, some by schools in Vietnam and others by the French Army in Indochina. They were generally dedicated to the French cause, highly reliable, and were fluent in the French language. Field duty was rotated among the staff as required by the circumstances.

The morning after we arrived, we attended a three-hour staff briefing. Normal duties at the hospital were set up and nurses were assigned on a rotating basis for floor duty. A pair of nurses, at least one legionnaire paramedic, and three Vietnamese paramedics worked in three, eight-hour shifts. At first, Margaret and I were assigned different hours. However, as often as we could, we changed shifts so we could work together. Change, a new experience in a new place, always made life more interesting and I enjoyed it.

However, Dr. Boof, a newly arrived surgeon from Cap St. Jacques, reiterated Dr. Carpentier's warnings about escalated fighting in our area. At night, the Viet Minh were attacking Hue and the surrounding villages with greater regularity. He warned us to be off the streets by eight o'clock.

Unlike at the Tourane hospital, we treated civilians, primarily indigenous personnel, at Hue. We saw many cases of malaria and dysentery caused by the overall unsanitary conditions within the area. One day, I came to work to find a five-year-old Vietnamese girl waiting for treatment. She looked pregnant because her stomach, as hard as a rock, protruded. I examined her and determined she probably had beriberi. I immediately called Dr. Seuzier and he verified my diagnosis. Beriberi is caused by a lack of vitamin B and is characterized by neuritis, often with muscle atrophy, poor coordination, and eventually by paralysis. Death often follows by heart failure. The disease is especially prevalent in those parts of the east where the diet consists mainly of polished rice. If the disease is caught early enough, recovery is prompt when adequate amounts of vitamin B-1 are restored to the diet. However, our little patient's coordination was all but gone and she was almost paralyzed. Dr. Seuzier ordered an IV for her and a heavy shot of vitamin B-1, but her disease had progressed too far and she died the same evening. Margaret and I went to the chapel after finishing our shift and prayed for her.

I eagerly looked forward each day to mail delivery, but to my dismay, I had not received mail from Maman or Suzanne since before Christmas. Their letters represented my connection to home, and I always worried when I did not hear from them.

On January 20, 1952, I became sick and was unable to go to work. The next morning when Margaret returned from her shift, she found me unconscious on the bathroom floor. She called the ambulance and I was taken to the emergency room. Dr. Seuzier diagnosed acute dysentery. Margaret told him about our oyster-induced episode in December. He said that the disease often recurred and gave me a shot of emetine and sulfa capsules. Dr. and Mrs. Carlson visited me everyday. They always brought flowers and talked to me about Minnesota. I began to feel better within a week, but I stayed in the hospital for 10 days before I was released.

 I returned to my quarters the first week in February and stayed there for a few days before returning to work. Dr. Seuzier cautioned me to eat very carefully and ensure my food had been properly disinfected. The Carlsons came to visit me each day and we became good friends. They were the kindest people I had ever met. I adored both of them and they treated me more like a daughter than the stranger I really was. It seemed they had decided to informally adopt both Margaret and me.

 Ruth, in particular, was a godsend. I was very weak and depressed when I was first released from the hospital. I confided to her my problems with Roger and my feelings about divorce. She told me that divorcing Roger was the right thing to do. "You never had a real marriage with him." She also comforted me about not receiving mail from Maman or Suzanne. Ruth told me not to worry because sometimes she did not receive mail from her children for four or six months, then she would get it all at once. Her upbeat attitude helped my mental state immensely which also helped me regain my physical strength.

 When I reported back to work I was feeling better, but my weight had dropped to 85 pounds and I was still weak. As I completed rounds that evening, I visited with a French captain who was recovering from a chest wound. He told me that he had been in Indochina for seven months and was also a veteran of World War II. "In all that time," he told me, "I had never been so discouraged; the enemy here in Vietnam is almost phantom-like. I have seldom seen the Viet Minh. We only react to their ambushes. So many times my troops have been killed by unseen snipers, booby traps, or land mines. It is such a different war." He lamented, "Although many of the Vietnamese seem loyal to us, you never really know if their loyalty is genuine. One of my patrols killed a sniper and after bringing his body to Hue, we found out that he had worked for the French government for more than five years—a supposed French loyalist!" He also believed that the Catholic Vietnamese were much more loyal to the French cause than the rest of the population because they were convinced the communists would eliminate religion if they ever gained full control of Vietnam.[12] He thought we could win the war with the Viet Minh if the French government would supply the personnel and supplies needed. His primary fear was that, because of all the political and economic troubles in France, the government would never prioritize the French presence in Indochina and that we would lose the colony. I thanked him for speaking to me about the situation and continued my rounds. His sincerity and concerns about our continued presence in Indochina worried me. It was incomprehensible to me how a small contingent of Viet Minh could defeat a powerful nation, least of all my beloved France.

The Carlsons loved Vietnam and its people. During the week, they visited the parishioners of the church and also the civilian and military hospitals in Hue. After seeing us working everyday when they visited the hospital and comforting me when I was sick in January, Margaret and I felt very close to the Carlsons. So when they invited us to attend church with them, we eagerly accepted. Though the northeast monsoon was still lingering past the season, Margaret and I put on our best dresses, carried our umbrellas, and met them at the Christian Church. They introduced us to their friends. Except for the Carlsons, Margaret, and I, only two other Caucasians were in the church. Mrs. Carlson played the piano and we especially enjoyed the choir.

I had never attended a Protestant service before and found it much different from Catholic mass which was then conducted in Latin. Pastor Carlson gave a beautiful sermon. He spoke on the unity of family and friends. He stressed the hopelessness brought upon the population by the divisive forces within Indochina: "The Indochinese and the French must find ways, other than armed conflict, to resolve their differences." He was an excellent preacher and spoke French like a native. It was an inspiring speech and he gave me hope that I would someday find true love and be happy.

As we were leaving the church, Dr. Carlson and his wife asked us to have lunch in their home. The maid first served us a salad with a tangy oil and vinegar dressing. It was delicious; however, I was not accustomed to eating salad as the first course. The French generally eat salad at the end of the meal. The main course was a beef stew with small new potatoes. It was served with JELL-0® on the side. Margaret and I had never seen or eaten JELL-0® before (a fact which amazed Mrs. Carlson), but we found the sweet jiggling substance quite good. We had napoleons for dessert with French coffee. It was an excellent meal and Margaret and I stuffed ourselves on what was our first home-cooked American meal.

After lunch, we retired to the living room where the Carlsons showed us slides of America for more than three hours, including numerous pictures of her two sons. One son was a minister and the other was in medical school. They encouraged us to visit America after we completed our tour in Indochina and gave us their American address and that of their sons. They also suggested that we learn at least conversational-level English. They drove us back to the house late in the afternoon and invited us to come by whenever we had time off from work. Margaret and I spent the remainder of the evening at home listening to music and talking about our futures. My dreams became increasingly entwined with visions of America.

We had been assigned the morning shift and our hopeful mood was dashed when we arrived at the hospital. The wards were full of patients. During the night, the Viet Minh had completely burned a small village near Hue. Much of the population had been burned or injured during the fighting. Although we were not equipped to properly treat burn injuries, we did the best we could with the medications on hand. The Viet Minh were becoming much bolder in their resistance and violently punishing French-loyalist Vietnamese. We worked all day and night, until three o'clock the next morning, stabilizing our patients. We went home exhausted and depressed. It seemed so futile. I remembered Dr. Carlson's sermon on unity and wondered if Indochina would ever achieve the peace and freedom he had so elegantly described. Margaret and I sat down on our porch, trying to settle our nerves, and drank cafe au lait. Margaret was happy that she would be leaving soon which depressed me even more. It seemed I was always losing my best friends.

We woke up early the next morning and took a long walk along the Perfume River where many children played and washed in the filthy, smelly water. We would never have dreamed of swimming in the polluted Vietnamese rivers, but many fishermen and their families lived in their boats, bathing and drinking the river water. The riverfront was always busy during the daylight hours. Numerous sampans delivered food and goods to the merchants in the area. People sat on their haunches over fish-filled baskets chanting the prices of their goods like auctioneers. We were always amazed at how cheerful and happy the Vietnamese people seemed. As we walked, many smiled and greeted us, some in French, but most in the Vietnamese language. We had learned a few words of Vietnamese, especially phrases of greeting and farewell and we could ask how a soldier felt or where it hurt. Most Vietnamese could interpret our pathetic attempts to speak their language. The French language was taught in all the Indochinese primary, secondary, and postsecondary schools.

As I watched the bustle of the marketplace, I could not help thinking that most of the people I saw were just like those we had treated in the hospital the day before. They were trying to make a living and raise their families. I wondered if the Viet Minh that burned the villagers yesterday would victimize these riverfront people tomorrow.

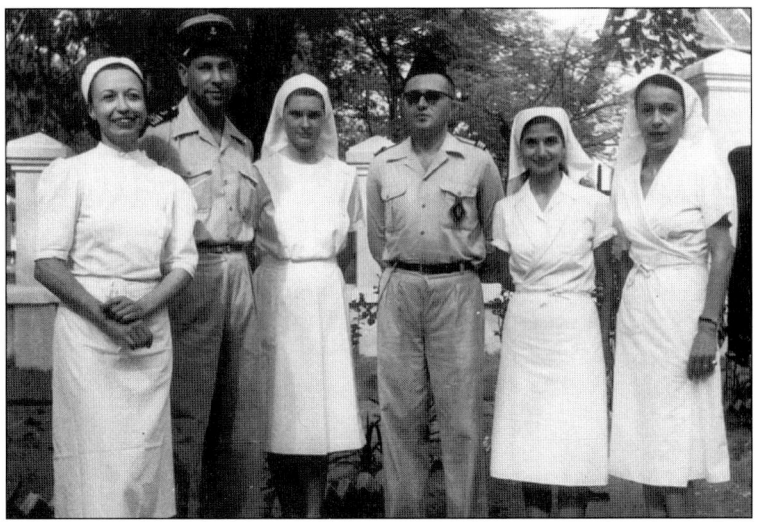

Danielle, Dr. Lariat, Janine, Dr. Mattei, Elisabeth, Denise

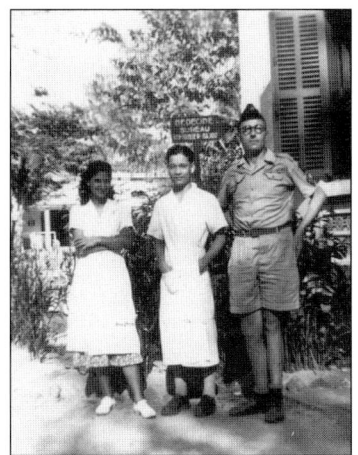

Elisabeth with paramedics

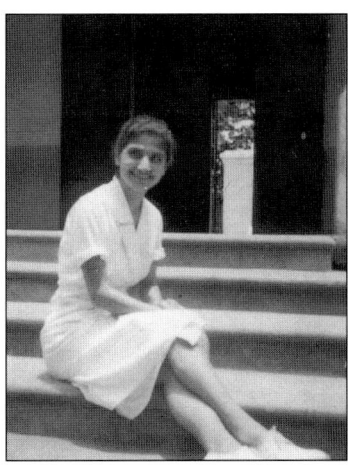

Elisabeth at Hue hospital

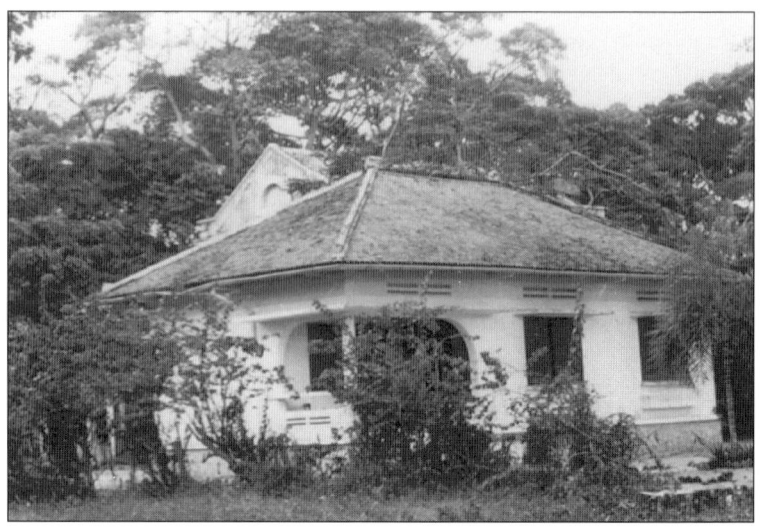
Home at Hue

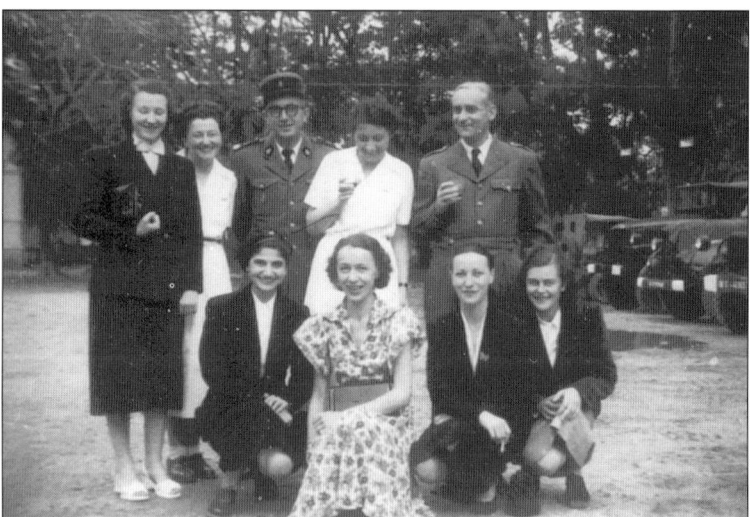
Crew at Hue

Chapter 6
Mouse Trapped

"*E*lisabeth, there is a gentleman in the office who claims to be your husband," the young paramedic announced.

"Tell him that I won't be available for another two or three hours." I hoped Roger would leave and not come back.

I was very busy in the ward. After two hours of treating incoming wounded, I reluctantly went to my office. Roger was still there, sitting in my chair. He greeted me with: "You've lost a lot of weight." He also told me that Paula had promised to marry him as soon as he returned from Indochina. He brought back a flood of bad memories and again I felt rejected. He gave me a letter from Paula that stated her undying love for him. "You can forward that to your lawyer to expedite our divorce." Then Roger informed me that he was assigned to the Hue garrison which did not help my morale.

During the first week of March, we received word that a Viet Minh battalion was concentrated near Quang Tri and presumably would be making a concerted effort to take over the city. Drs. Lariat and Mattei were being transferred from Tourane to join our staff. We had also received two new nurses, Janine, just out of school in France, and Yvette, a transfer from Tourane. Our casualties began to increase dramatically as our patrols engaged the enemy on a daily basis. We learned that an entire patrol had been ambushed and everyone had been killed or taken prisoner. Dr. Mattei asked for volunteers to go to Quang Tri and set up a triage station. Drs. Deit, Boof, Seuzier were going. Margaret, Janine, and I immediately volunteered. We were the youngest nurses, unattached, and still foolish enough to believe we were immortal.

Within the week, we left by convoy with a French battalion going to reinforce the company in Quang Tri. The legionnaires were able to set up our entire site in less than three hours. We were better equipped than when we had operated near the same area in 1951. We even had two gasoline generators to supply electrical power, three small airplanes to take the critically wounded to Hue, and much more modern (American) medical equipment. To my surprise, 15 American soldiers were serving as advisors to the French forces. I was impressed with the Americans' friendliness, optimism, and self-assurance.

I invited a sergeant into our operating tent for a cup of coffee. "Are the Americans going to join us in the fight against the Viet Minh?"

"We're only here as advisors. We can't take part in the actual combat."

After we shared with him our hope that the French could keep the communists from taking over Vietnam, he continued, "Frankly, I hope that we do not take up the battle in Indochina if the French should leave. It's important to help our allies, but I don't think America has any real purpose or mission in Indochina."

I felt safe with so many soldiers around us and I went to sleep early. I was awakened by the sound of artillery shells at three o'clock in the morning. I got up very fast and had coffee to settle my nerves. I looked at the men in the lookout tower. They were still there but evidently no one knew from which direction the shells were coming. Dr. Mattei went to battalion headquarters, a local farmhouse, to see what was happening. He found out that our patrols had been ambushed and we would soon be receiving wounded. The paramedics were assigned to help Dr. Boof in triage while each nurse was assigned to assist Drs. Mattei and Deit in surgery.

In less than two hours we received our first patients. I could tell by their wounds—many needed amputations—that the fighting had been intense. According to our men, the problem was the same: They had been on patrol looking for the Viet Minh, but could never see or hear them. Then, all of a sudden, there was gunfire and they found themselves surrounded by the enemy. When they moved out, they came upon carefully placed minefields or booby traps which took a great toll upon them. The worst cases were airlifted to Hue and the others were sent by ambulance to either Tourane or Hue.

I distinctly remember a young patient named Martin. He had stepped on a mine and Dr. Mattei took two hours to remove his legs. After the surgery, Dr. Mattei asked me to suture the severed limbs, because he desperately needed to take care of another patient. It seemed the floor of the operating tent was a river of blood during the entire engagement.

The first day we worked from six o'clock in the morning until after dark. It was impossible for the autoclave to keep up with the need for sterilized equipment; therefore, we washed the instruments in alcohol and let them air dry. Late that night, after treating 80 patients, our load became slower and we could take turns resting for a few hours. The medical team probably only slept an average of three to four hours each day during the battle. I worked one stretch of more than 36 hours before being relieved. The surgeons probably only slept an average of two to three hours each day.

During the first week, we also had 20 wounded Viet Minh prisoners brought in for treatment. We took care of their injuries begrudgingly; during the first week, the French battalion had lost more than 200 personnel by death or injury. The second week the French battalion received reinforcements to replace the wounded.

At the beginning of the third week at Quang Tri, we had a short respite. We used the time to sleep but some members of the medical team were so distressed by the carnage that they found it impossible to rest for very long. I slept for six hours, then played cards to forget the war, killing, and agony I had witnessed. Unfortunately, the lull in action was not to last. As we were playing cards, a messenger passed an envelope to Dr. Mattei who read the note and summoned the rest of the team. He announced, "The reason we haven't seen much action the past 12 hours is because we're totally encircled by the Viet Minh. It will probably be only a matter of hours before they attack in full force. Let's hope that reinforcements from Hue can get here in time." He then gave each of the nurses cyanide pills to take if we were captured. The merciless Viet Minh would spare the women no torture or humiliation if they caught us alive.

Shortly after our meeting, I developed a fever of more than 104 degrees. I was delirious and did not know what was going on. Dr. Mattei took a sample of my blood and determined I was suffering from *falciparum* (malignant) malaria.[13] He immediately began giving me huge doses of quinine and nivaquine. I was in and out of consciousness for the next seven days, only remembering the doctor saying, "She's probably not going to make it."

I was also hallucinating, but one day felt a new kind of pain in my feet. I managed to focus on three rabbit-sized, foul-smelling rats gnawing on my feet. My adrenaline really woke me up and I kicked the nasty beasts off of me. I screamed and the staff immediately came to check me. Dr. Mattei wanted to give me a morphine shot, but I would not take it because I was afraid I would not be able to fend off the rodents if I was sedated. Later I realized that the rats saved my life. They forced me into consciously fighting to survive. I slowly regained my strength and my fever subsided.

After I was strong enough to ask, I learned that the French battalion from Hue, led by Major Marcel Madec, had broken through the Viet Minh lines and rescued us. Though more than 200 Viet Minh prisoners were captured and sent to camps in southern Vietnam, the French lost more personnel in this battle than in any other up to that time in Vietnam. When our convoy returned to Hue, the streets were packed with people, and the battalion band played and led us into the garrison. The French commander had set up a parade as we reentered the city. It was a heartwarming experience for all of us.

When we arrived at our base, Major Madec and I were escorted to the front of the formation and Major Madec was presented the Croix de Guerre, and I was presented the Medaille Coloniale. We were both very happy about the honors bestowed upon us.

The commander at Hue scheduled a big homecoming celebration at the Officers' Club for the weekend. Margaret, Janine, and I eagerly prepared for the big celebration. We bought new formal dresses for the occasion. I chose a white, full-length gown that accentuated my complexion. Since I only weighed 80 pounds, I had a dressmaker tailor mine to fit. We also bought new shoes and accessories. Like young school girls going to our first prom, on the day of the party we had our hair done, nails manicured, and eyes made up.

Dr. Mattei had arranged for all the nurses to be picked up by automobile and taken to the Officers' Club. We arrived a few minutes after eight o'clock in the evening and were seated at four-person tables. Margaret and I were joined by Dr. Lariat and Major Madec.

I was thrilled to be sitting with Major Madec, the savior of our battalion. He was good looking: 40 years old, around 5 feet

10 inches tall, somewhat stocky, and had brown hair and hazel eyes. He had been in Indochina for two years and had been a battalion commander for two months. Most of his men were French Moroccans who were renowned for their fierce fighting abilities. Major Madec was an unmarried graduate of St. Cyr, the West Point of France, and was from Bretagne, which is northwest of Paris. We talked about our families and our various duties in Indochina. After dinner, the brigadier general in charge of the Hue garrison made a toast to Major Madec and thanked him for his courageous breakthrough to relieve our troops.

After dinner, the band arrived and played all the old French songs. It was grand. Dr. Lariat and I danced until someone cut in. I must have danced with six or seven different partners, including Major Madec and Dr. Mattei, and did not get back to the table until the band stopped for a break. It was a beautiful evening and I was sorry when it ended at midnight. We were taken by automobile back to our quarters and Margaret and I sat up for two more hours talking about the wonderful time we had dancing and the different people we had met.

During the second week of April, I received a letter from my lawyer in Tourane informing me that my divorce from Roger was final on March 14, 1952. I was glad that Roger was finally out of my life forever.

Margaret left Indochina at the end of April and I felt as lonely as I had ever been. Living alone in the house added to my depression. I also received a shocking letter from Suzanne. She informed me that she had "met a good friend of mine," the paramedic who had stolen her photograph. He had written her and when he returned to France, they started dating. "It was a whirlwind romance," she wrote and then dropped the bomb: She had married him! She stated Maman was happy about her marriage, but I was devastated. I knew his reputation, and he clearly was unsuitable marriage material for my sister. I knew the marriage would never last and felt Suzanne would be in for much suffering before it was over. However, there was nothing I could do except pray for her. I felt guilty because it was my carelessness that had enabled the rogue to obtain Suzanne's address. Being so far away from home, not being there to protect Suzanne, made me feel even more isolated in Indochina.

However, the Carlsons always had time for me and they welcomed me to their home for visits and meals. I also spent some time with Major Madec whenever he was in Hue. We usually went to the Officers' Club for dinner and then walked and talked. We really became quite good friends and he cheered me up considerably. I was worried about his safety because I knew the war was being accelerated and I hoped and prayed he would make it through unscathed, so I was pleased and relieved that he wrote frequently when he was away from Hue.

We had many wounded patients from the Quang Tri battle still in the ward. Though most were recovering, a few remained in precarious health. One of my chest-wound patients wanted water but was not allowed anything to drink. While a paramedic was changing the bottles from the drain tubes in the patient's chest, the wounded man screamed in pain and I moistened his burning lips and parched tongue. "My chest is on fire," he cried. He calmed down when I explained that water would only create more fluid on his lungs, but I'll never forget the despair on his face as he murmured, "I want to die."

Dr. Boof agreed that I should give him morphine. After administering the shot, I continued my rounds and counted six patients with serious chest wounds. I kept moistening their lips and ensuring that they received morphine when they needed it. One patient, next to the wall at the end of the hall, was stretched out and in a delirious state. A paramedic had to hold him down while he cried out to his mother loudly and incoherently. He had malaria and his bed was soaked in his own sweat. My mind went back to my recent bout with malaria and I wondered if I had perspired so much. I gave him a shot of morphine to calm him down.

When I had been in the ballroom dancing the night before, I had not thought of my patients and upon returning to the hospital, I felt guilty for enjoying myself while these brave men were suffering so much. I also missed Margaret. My heart was broken and I was overwhelmed with all the suffering around me. I felt inadequate because there was so little I could do to help them. Many of my patients would die while others would take months or even years to heal. For only the second time in my military career, I wanted to go home.

I was shaken from my thoughts when the paramedic called me to the bedside of the patient I had tended earlier in the morning. His drainage bottle was filling with blood. I called Dr. Mattei immediately and then began to scream in my frustration. His face was contorted with pain. I knew he was dying—I had seen the death look innumerable times. His glassy eyes were fixed on my face as he begged for water. A great determination came over me and I poured a glass of water and held it to his lips. He feverishly drank one-half of the water before his head sank back, his eyes closed, and he breathed a long sigh. He died in peace. I was frozen in place and Dr. Mattei shook his head and then took my arm. "Such a waste," he said. He took me to the break room and consoled me. After Dr. Mattei left, I went outside to get some fresh air and compose myself. I could not feel sorry for myself for long as I had many more patients who needed my help. So I prayed I would not lose more patients, shook my head, and went back to work. I was at peace with myself and my duties became my challenge.

A few days later, two of my patients had recovered to the point where we could give them water to drink. I was so proud of them and my morale increased upon seeing them getting along so well. Within a week, the tubes of the chest patients were removed and they were walking with the help of the paramedics.

Evidently, God had answered my prayers because I did not lose another patient from the March 1952 Quang Tri battle.

When Major Madec took three days off to visit Tourane, he asked me to accompany him. I requested a three-day pass that Dr. Mattei enthusiastically approved, "You need to get away from it all and rejuvenate your soul." Then he added, "But come back like the old Elisabeth." Exuberant and with my energy restored, I happily told Major Madec that I would be free to join him. My spirits immediately rose.

Major Madec picked me up after work on Friday and we drove in his jeep to Tourane. My old friends in Tourane did not know that I was coming and they were surprised and happy to see me when I arrived. I slept in the hospital and Major Madec stayed in the officer's quarters on post. Dr. Lariat insisted on taking us to dinner. We went to a small restaurant owned by a Frenchman who had been born in Indochina. He had a beautiful concubine, a Eurasian girl. After a warm welcome, they prepared a special French meal for us. We had a wonderful dinner with white wine and then sat around and talked over cafe au lait. Dr. Lariat told me he was probably going to be transferred to Hue. I hoped he would join our staff because I really liked and respected him.

During dinner, Dr. Lariat told us how Tourane was becoming a stronghold for the Viet Minh. They had terrorized the city several times within the past two months. Major Madec was well aware of the buildup of the Viet Minh in the central plains of Vietnam. His battalion was experiencing more resistance each passing day.

We began to reminisce about our younger days in France. I told them about my school days in convents and experiences in the Resistance. Our conversation turned to our hopes for after the war. Dr. Lariat told me his wife had contracted a severe case of acute dysentery and had been repatriated to La Martinique. She was doing fine and he was looking forward to rejoining her and their two children. Major Madec's mother had been diagnosed with cancer and he hoped to get back to France to spend time with her and his father. We finally ran out of talk and left to go back to our quarters.

The next day, we went to the Museum of Cham Sculpture in Tourane.[14] The museum was set up in 1936 by the *Ecole Francaise d'Extreme Orient*. The culture and history of the Cham people are revealed through their sculptures and carvings. We toured the museum all morning, had a light lunch, and then departed for the Marble Mountains, also known as the Mountains of the Five Elements. We visited the Tam Thi Temple, the Linh Ung Temple, and Huyen Khong Grotto. The mountains are a valuable source of red, white, and blue-green marble which was used by the local population to chisel out a great variety of *Objects d'art*. It was late afternoon before we completed our tour and returned to Tourane.

We rested at the hospital for a couple of hours before going out with some of the hospital staff to our favorite French restaurant downtown. It was so good to get away from the stress and sadness of the war for just a few hours. I returned to the hospital and went to sleep feeling relaxed and happy to have spent some time with friends.

Major Madec picked me up about noon the next day and we returned to Hue. I told him how much I had enjoyed our few days together. He had become such a good friend, I could tell him anything without worrying about him repeating it. He was a man of honor and someone I respected completely. I felt fortunate in being his friend and confidante. His friendship meant so much to me because he was so much like Papa. He had become the father figure I had so much missed since Papa had been killed early in World War II.

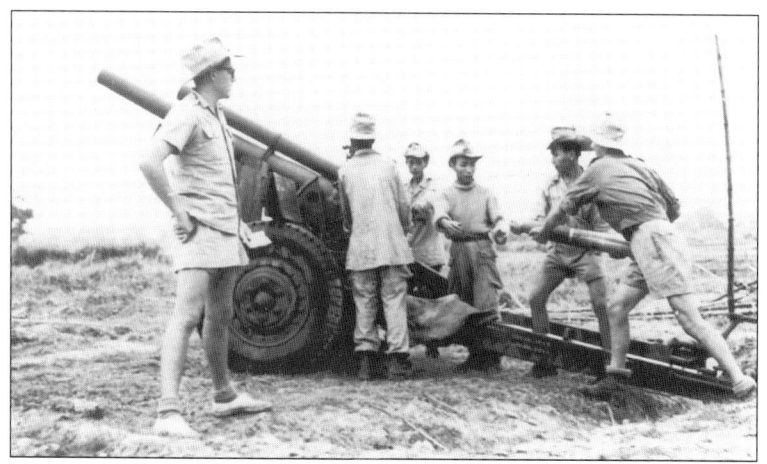

Artillery unit — Quang Tri

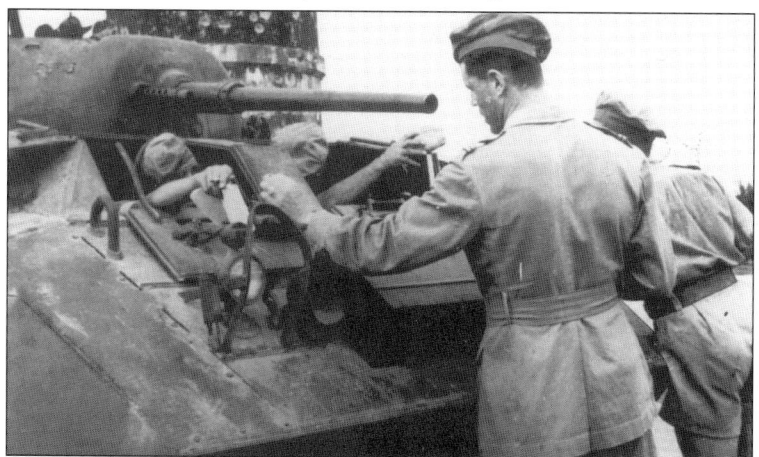

French tank at Quang Tri

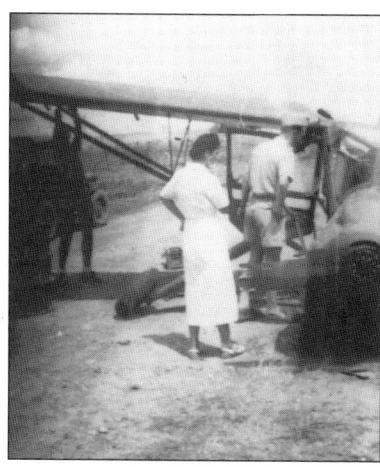

Medical evacuation airplane

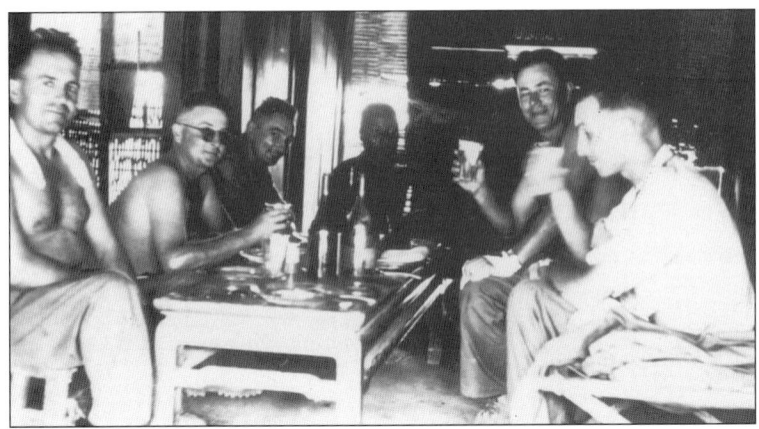
Major Madec with his officers

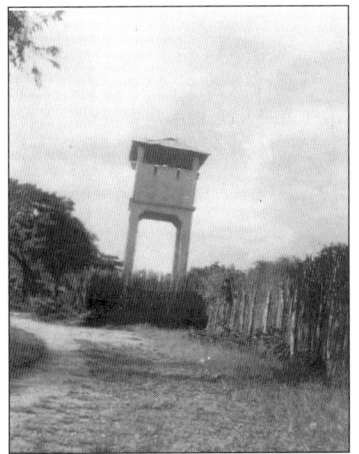
Lookout tower — Quang Tri

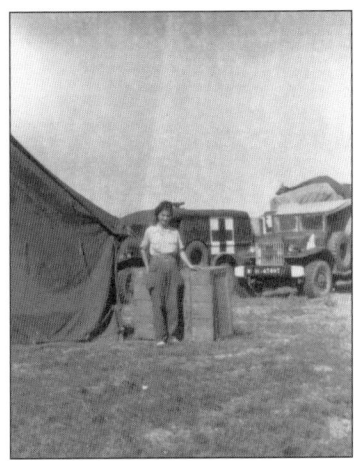
Medical tent near Quang Tri

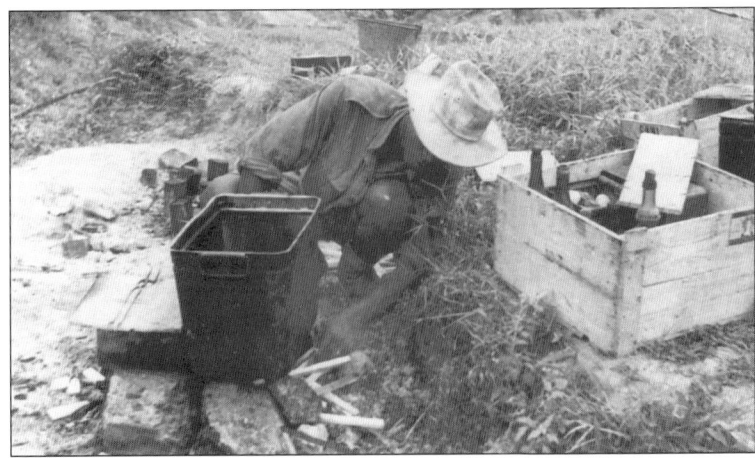
Cook setting up for coffee

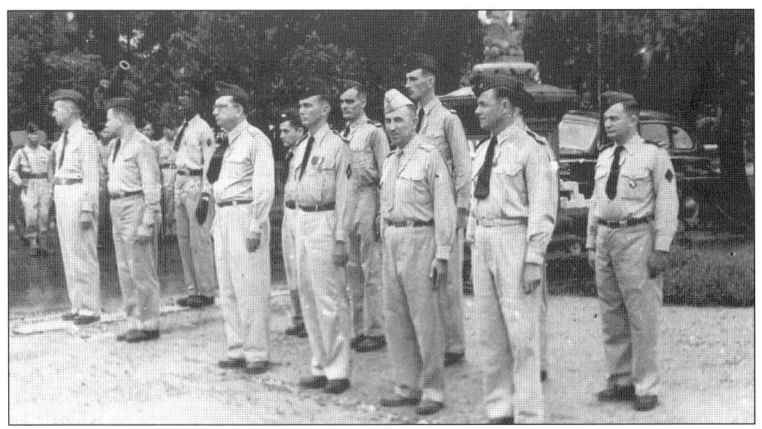

Major Madec (front right) receiving award

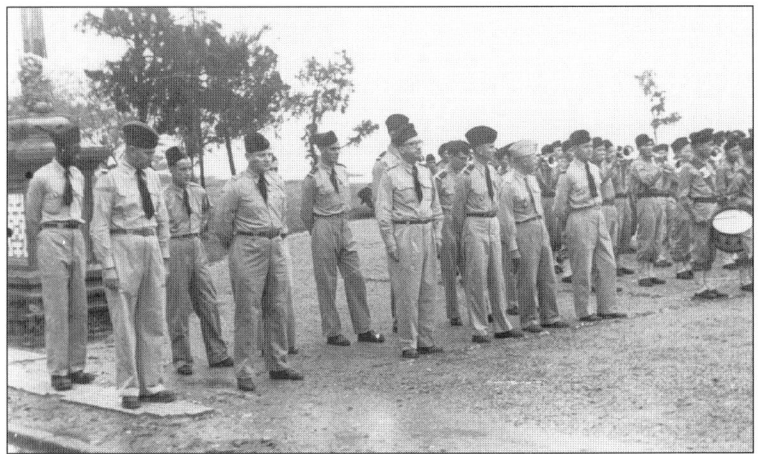

Parade in Hue

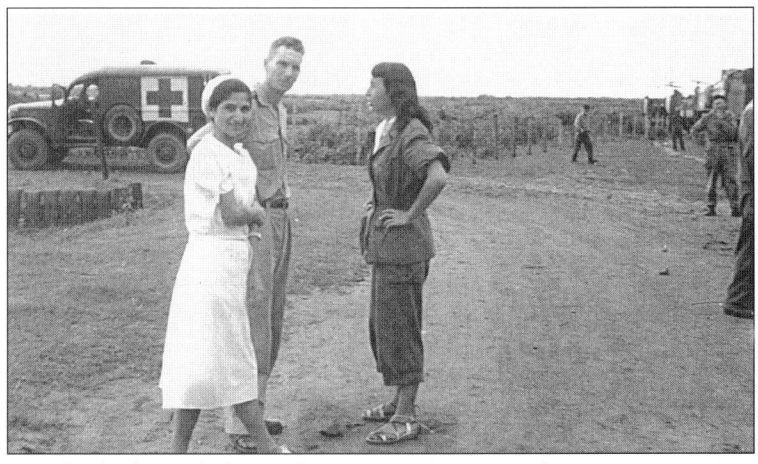

Elisabeth, ambulance driver, French paramedic in Quang Tri

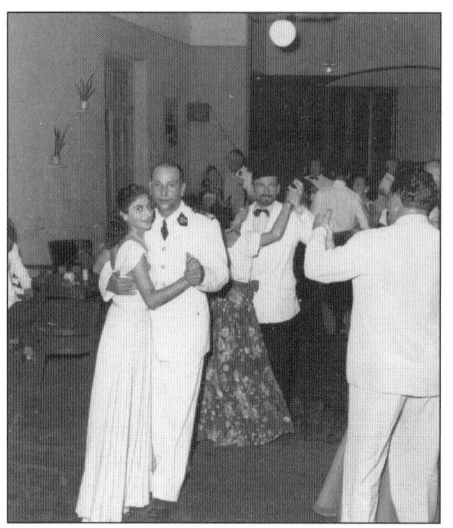
Officers' Club — Hue

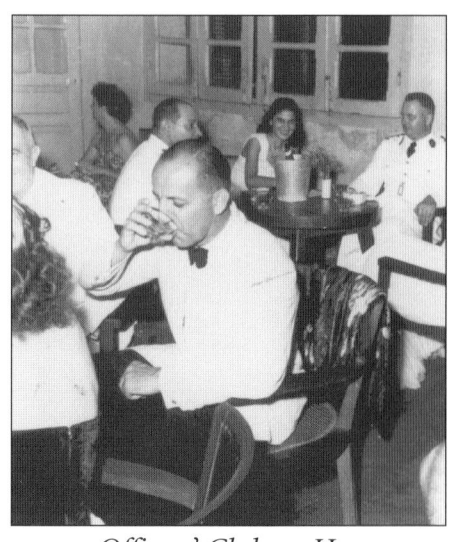
Officers' Club — Hue

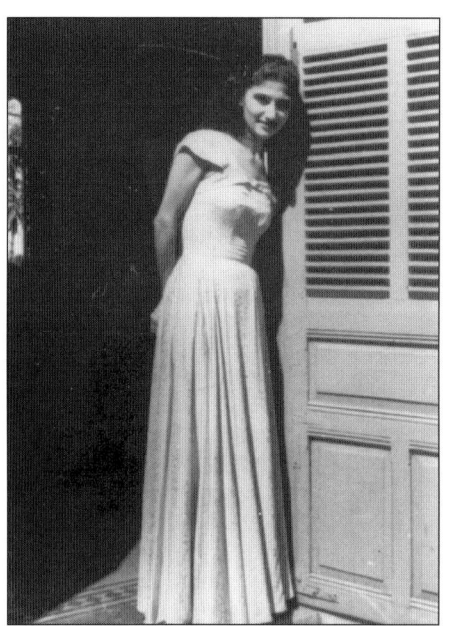
Elisabeth's party dress

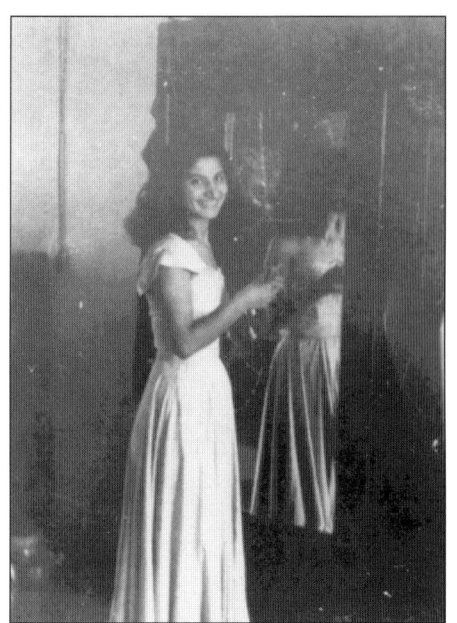
Dressing for party

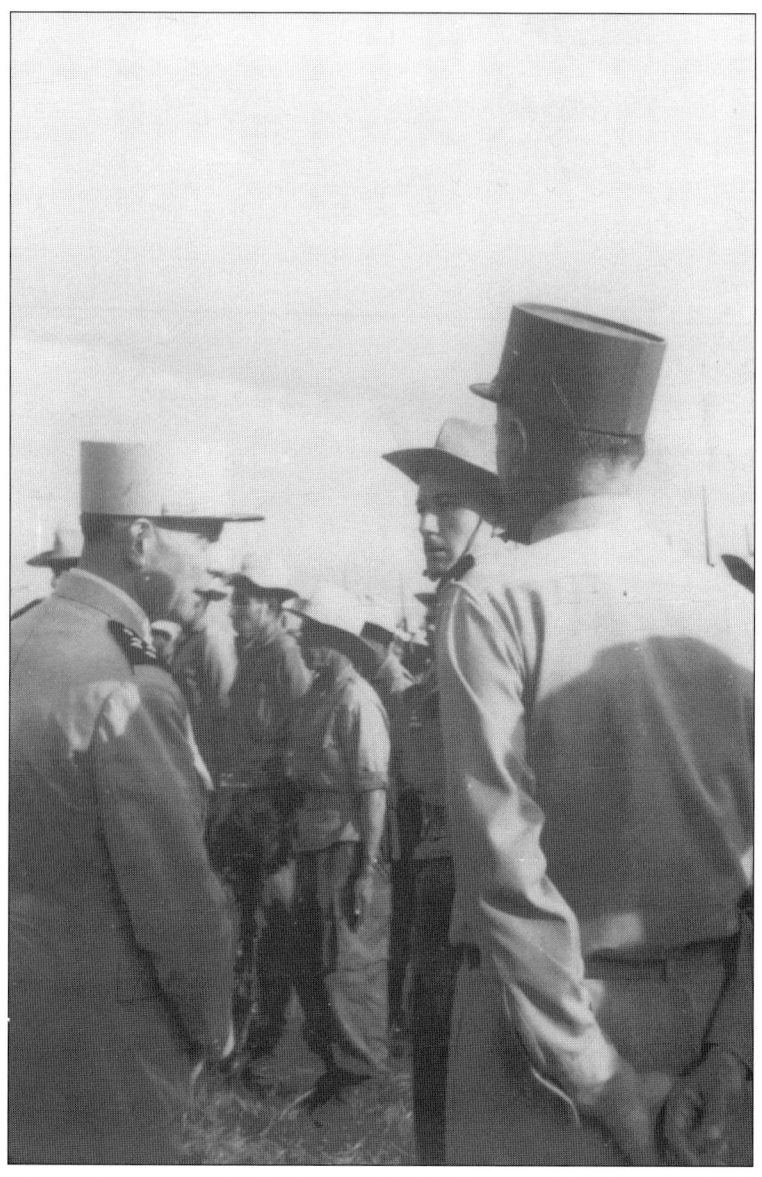

General de Lattre de Tassigny with Philippe, a friend of Elisabeth

Elisabeth Sevier with Robert Sevier

Chapter 7
Laos

I went back to work refreshed and happy. I was thrilled that Janine had decided to move into the house with me. We got along very well and she had become my best friend since Margaret left. Since Janine had also taken over Margaret's assignment, it was very easy for us to live and work together.

The hospital was almost full with many cases of malaria and dysentery. The week went smoothly and I was able to spend a couple of evenings with the Carlsons. They always seemed happy to receive me. Again we viewed color slides of the United States, including those of the Grand Canyon, Yellowstone Park, Mount Rushmore, and the Grand Teton Mountains. They also had slides of Salt Lake City, the Mormon Tabernacle, and the Great Salt Lake. My fascination with the States, especially after meeting other Americans while in the field, grew. It seemed a magical place: so large, so varied a population, and such beautiful scenery.

At the beginning of June 1952, we received word that the Viet Minh were building up their forces in Laos, a French protectorate.[15] Within a week, we moved into Laos to set up an aid station. Major Madec's battalion was also deployed to the area; therefore, I felt safe. The medical detachment consisted of Drs. Mattei and Boof as well as Janine, a new nurse, Dominique, and me.

The trip through the mountains seemed to go on forever. The heat was suffocating and the humidity was always near 100 percent. During the southwest monsoon season, which lasted from May to October, it rained incessantly and the days were extremely hot and humid. Most of the population lived in the lowlands where the principal products were coffee and rice. Because of the flash flooding caused by excessive rainfall, all the houses were built on pillars that stood about one and one-half meters high. I noticed the women were taller than those of Vietnam and wore colorful homespun skirts.

We stopped near the village of Muang Xepon, which is 100 kilometers due west from Quang Tri, and set up our aid station seven kilometers from the town. The paramedics quickly put up our tents while the soldiers erected a lookout tower. That evening, Major Madec stopped by to speak to our doctors. He had sent three patrols out to check the area and all the patrols had returned without seeing any Viet Minh. The evening and the next day were quiet. We rested and played cards to pass the time.

About noon on the third day, a message came in from the chief of Muang Xepon informing us the Viet Minh had raided the town during the night and taken all the young village males. The chief was scared that they would return to destroy the town, so Major Madec sent a company of Moroccans to fortify it. The Viet Minh returned that evening and during the skirmish killed a dozen Moroccans. A number of injured soldiers and some of the village inhabitants were brought into our aid station for treatment. We shipped the more seriously wounded by airplane to Hue.

The following two days were very quiet, and our troops did not encounter any of the Viet Minh. However, at five o'clock the next afternoon, the Viet Minh attacked with mortars and artillery. We responded with our own artillery and patrols. The conflict lasted five days and our aid station was swamped with both wounded soldiers and civilians.

Most of the time, we worked day and night, only sleeping when one could no longer function. The doctors were so busy that we had to bring them portable urinals so they could relieve themselves without stopping their operations. They were completely exhausted but somehow managed to handle the medical situation. After five days, our troops successfully drove off the invading Viet Minh. Both sides had experienced heavy losses, but the French had survived their strongest attacks and gave them more than they received. However, Maung Xepon had been destroyed. We were busy the next few days stabilizing our patients and getting them ready for transport to Hue. Our efforts were compounded by the southwest monsoon. It rained both day and night, only letting up for brief periods.

Heartsick over the losses of French-loyalist Laotians, I was depressed and felt dirty. We had not showered since leaving Hue. Janine and I located two large buckets, made holes in the bottom of one, and collected rainwater in the other. Then we cut four large bamboo stalks and located two army blankets. We took all of our homemade gear into the trees where we stuck the bamboo stalks into the ground and draped the blankets. I took off my clothes in our primitive shelter while Janine sat in the small tree with the two buckets. When I was ready, she poured some rainwater into the holey bucket and I had a shower I will always remember. We traded places and Janine took her shower while I emptied the bucket above her. Just as we were finishing, we heard several voices. Three paramedics, who had been sent out by Dr. Boof to find us, laughed like crazy when they spotted us in our jerry-built shower. We finished dressing into our dirty clothes and accompanied them back to the aid station. Drs. Boof and Mattei were greatly disturbed by our escapade. "Don't even think of doing something like that again! We're in combat here."

The next morning, we loaded up our trucks and departed for Quang Tri where we took the train to Hue. The train was relatively new, built expressly for use by the French military. We got back to Hue with all 82 of our patients in fairly good shape. Dr. Lariat, who had transferred to Hue while we were in Laos, picked us up at the station. Seeing him and the sunshine improved my morale. He gave us the day off and I went home to enjoy a long hot bath, clean clothes, and some much needed sleep.

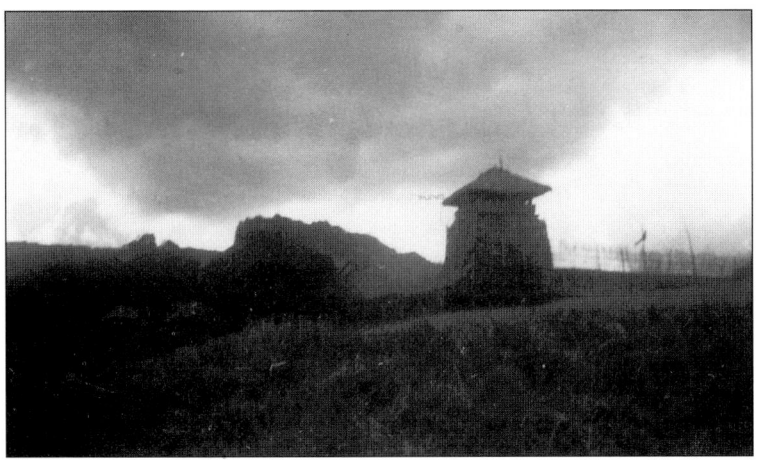
Lookout tower — Laos

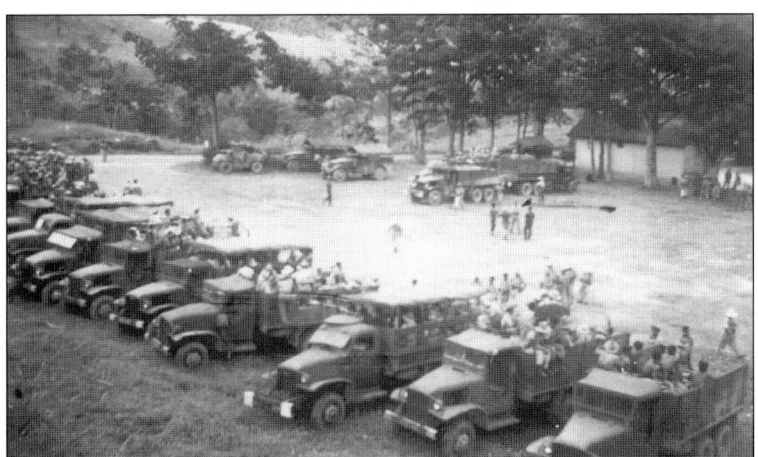
On the road to Laos

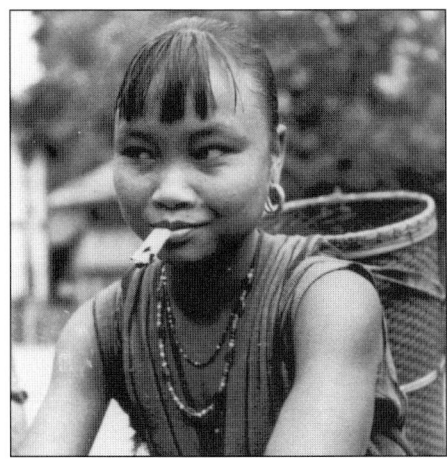
Young Laotian woman

Chapter 8
Rest and Relaxation

*J*anine and I slept very well during the night and returned to the hospital the next morning relaxed and ready to go back to work. As usual we attended the morning briefing and then began tending to our Laotian patients. We worked all day long and the time passed quickly.

However, time was passing very slowly for Dr. Lariat. He missed his family, but was denied permission for a two-week leave. The fighting was escalating and a replacement for him was not available. The general unpopularity of the war and the many domestic problems of the post-War French government made recruitment of doctors for Indochina extremely difficult. To us, it seemed the French people had forsaken the spirit of freedom for the Indochinese people.

To cheer up Dr. Lariat, we planned a big party at a fancy French restaurant for his 45th birthday. We decided to present him with money instead of a gift. We all split the cost of his food. Everyone from the hospital staff was present, except those who were left on duty at the hospital. The other doctors had invited Dr. Lariat to dinner and he thought it was just a small get-together of physicians. When he arrived at the restaurant and saw all the people there to wish him well, he was pleasantly surprised. The dinner was superb with French dishes served in the French manner, including champagne, coq au vin, French bread, various vegetables, and chocolate mousse for dessert. We had hired a small band and we danced until midnight. Everyone had a wonderful time and we all forgot about the war for a short time. Dr. Lariat seemed to really appreciate our efforts.

The next day we went to work and began sending some of our wounded back to their companies. It was a sad experience because I knew they would probably come back, many with greater wounds than they had experienced to date. Also, many would die because French casualties were increasing as each day passed.

Despite the party, Janine and I were still war-weary. Our two-week request for R and R (rest and relaxation) was granted and we decided to go to Da Lat which we had heard was a beautiful city surrounded by majestic mountains. We left early the next week, flying in military aircraft from Hue to Da Lat. We stayed at a beautiful villa which was maintained by the Officers' Club. We had separate, large rooms with a lovely view of the mountains. It was so peaceful and fresh we felt young and giddy, pleased with our choice of destination. Our meals were prepared by a cook in the villa and our rooms were cleaned each day by a maid. We just rested and took in the scenery for the first two days, walking around the grounds, and eating and sleeping as we desired.

We were happy when two other nurses from Saigon, Paulette and Marie, arrived the next day. They had been in Saigon for a year and said that they envied our duty as colonial nurses in the field. However, after we explained our responsibilities and experiences, they decided they were better off where they were.

The day after they arrived, we took pedicabs to visit the Da Lat sights and explored the city. Our driver was a tour guide and took us to the more interesting places in the city. He told us Da Lat was called the "City of Eternal Spring." We learned that "Da" means "river" or "source" in reference to the Cam Ly River, and

"Lat" is the name of an ethnic minority living there. The city is situated among mountains, pine-clad hillsides, lakes, and forests on the Lam Vien Plateau. The average annual temperature is about 70 degrees. The fresh mountain air and tranquil beauty of the area attracted the French who developed the resort and built their holiday villas on the hillside. Da Lat was noted as a favorite destination for lovers and honeymooners and had, at one time, been projected to become the eventual capital of the Indochinese State Federation under the French.[16] (To us, it seemed like a Garden of Eden.)

The next day, we visited the old French Quarter near the bridge spanning the Cam Ly River and the Da Lat Catholic Cathedral named Nha Tho Con Ga, which was built in 1931. Its stained glass windows were made by Louis Balmet in Grenoble. When we went inside, the priest invited us to Sunday mass. He escorted us throughout the church explaining its significance and history. Before we left, he asked us to take confession and we all did, making us feel better about ourselves. We thanked him and returned on the following Sunday as we had promised.

Everyone was really feeling good, the visit to the church had helped our morale because we were all brought up in the Catholic faith. We looked for a restaurant with a view of the mountains and found a charming place in the French Quarter. We had an excellent meal at a moderate price and lingered for two hours and then drank coffee outside on the terrace. The fresh, cool air was so exhilarating that we sat outside and talked until almost dark and then we decided to walk along the river. We felt safe, talking about our childhoods in France, away from the horrors of the war. Eventually, we went back to the villa and went to bed.

We spent the next day at the market in downtown Da Lat. We primarily watched the people as they went about their daily business. They sold a great assortment of fruits and vegetables. The strawberries were particularly luscious and we all bought some to eat as we walked through the market. We also bought small jars of strawberry jam to take home with us. After seeing the market, we visited the summer residence of Vietnam's last Nguyen emperor, Bao Dai. His summer palace stood in a well-maintained park a few blocks from the Catholic Cathedral. After our tour of the ornate home, we returned to our rooms and rested until dinner. We stayed in the villa that evening, playing cards and listening to both French and Vietnamese records.

On Thursday we went to the Da Lat Ethnic Minority Museum in Lam Dong Province. The museum displayed beautiful traditional costumes and ornaments. I was especially impressed by the exquisite and large pieces of jade on exhibit. There were also various musical instruments on display. I was struck by the statue of a Hindu Goddess named Uma. When I looked at the figure, I felt it looked right back into my eyes. We finished our visit late in the afternoon and returned to our villa. We were all tired from our journey and retired early because the pedicab driver insisted that we see the Lake of Sorrows.

The lake, named Ho Than Tho in Vietnamese, was located five kilometers from Da Lat. A guide told us that the lake derived its name from the patriotism of a young couple. When the man had joined the resistance force against the Tsin invaders, the girl believed her beloved would be better able to serve his country without worrying about her. Consequently, she drowned herself in the lake to free him from further concern. It was a beautiful lake and we cried after the guide told us the story of its name.

After the tour, we went to eat in Da Lat. As we were ready to leave, a young French captain came to our table. He looked straight at me, "Do you remember me?" It took me a moment, but my memory registered and I realized it was Philippe, a young officer I had met in Saigon when Margaret and I first arrived in Indochina. We had talked with him during lunch at the Officers'

Club in Saigon for more than two hours during our first days in country. Philippe was tall, with prematurely thinning hair, and charismatic. He was 30 years old and had graduated from St. Cyr.

Philippe told us that he was assigned as a liaison officer for the Montagnards who were valiant allies in our fight with the Viet Minh. The Montagnards were mountain people residing in the central highlands. They detested the Vietnamese because they had been mistreated by them for many years; their primitive lifestyle had been prey to the wily political aims of the Vietnamese government. The Viet Minh had tried to use this animosity toward the loyalist Vietnamese and recruit the Montagnards to their communist cause. However, the Montagnard's natural distrust for all Vietnamese made them unlikely volunteers. France had taken advantage of their prejudices and sent officers to train Montagnards in the fight against the Viet Minh. Philippe was one of the young officers assigned to advise and train the Montagnards.

The strong and wiry mountain people knew every inch of their tribal lands and had a history as fierce warriors. When they exchanged their crossbows and other primitive weapons for rifles, the Montagnards developed into highly effective irregular troops. Philippe invited us to accompany him back to his base camp. Janine and I decided it would be an interesting experience and told him we would go.

The next day we left with Philippe in his jeep. When we arrived at a small mountain village, M'Drack, Janine and I both noticed that the village women wore shawls draped over the back of their heads. Their homes were primarily huts constructed of bamboo with thatch roofs; each hut had a small vegetable garden. Philippe took us inside a house that served as his office. He fitted both of us with copper bracelets, telling us that the Montagnards would recognize us as friends if we wore them, and then we met the village chief. He was dressed in native Montagnard attire: a long chemise with trousers to match.

Philippe translated our brief conversation of greetings. We ended our short visit with the chief and went to Philippe's home. After we were given something to eat, Philippe escorted us to rooms where we would sleep. We retired early in the evening because we were tired from the journey.

The next morning, we awoke and had tea with Philippe, who had been up since dawn. He told us he had arranged a tour through the village and school and the chief had planned a welcoming celebration for us the following day. The village had been built in a kind of circle with an open area in the middle used for community activities and ceremonies. We walked through the village with Philippe who seemed to know everyone by name. It was evident the people knew and respected Philippe.

We went to the school which had been set up by Philippe with the assistance of the French government. The students were excited to see their strange visitors and some even came by and touched us. The teacher was very proud because his curriculum included the French language. He directed the students in singing a French song for us. We sat and watched the instruction and then visited with the students during their recess period. Some of the older children came and spoke with us in nonfluent, but understandable, French. They seemed to be proud of their ability to speak our language. Philippe took us throughout the village and then drove the jeep into the surrounding mountains to show us the beauty of the land. It was calm and peaceful. The vegetation and flowers were as beautiful as any we had seen in Vietnam. We returned to Philippe's home late in the afternoon and took a short nap. Janine and I rustled up the ingredients to prepare Philippe dinner. We ended up making rice and chicken over an open fire. The meal turned out to be delicious and Philippe was happy to be a treated to home-cooked meal.

Over breakfast, Philippe advised us that the Montagnards expected us to try each dish served during the afternoon ceremony given in our honor; they would be insulted if we did not eat all of the food. He also gave us another copper necklace as a souvenir, which we gratefully accepted. The ceremony was held where the chief resided, in a village a few kilometers from M'Drack, at two o'clock. When we arrived, the Montagnards were assembled in anticipation of our arrival. We were given flowers and seated in front with Philippe and the chief. We were presented cooked rice by some village women and a local alcoholic drink. As we ate and drank, the villagers sang for us. When they finished their songs, all the men lined up single file, with Philippe in the middle. Each man took a rifle and fired at targets strung up in nearby trees. They were laughing and seemed to really enjoy shooting. When a target was hit by a participant, everyone gave their approval by loud shouting. The ceremony ended with each of the villagers coming by and shaking hands with us. They seemed to be very happy people, but extremely primitive and poor. We left the ceremony at its end and returned to Philippe's hut. The drinks had made Janine and I so drowsy that we slept immediately and did not wake up until the next morning.

The next day Philippe drove us back to Tourane where we caught the train to Hue. I appreciated the opportunity Philippe had given us to see the Montagnard culture. It had been an interesting and unique three days.

Elisabeth Sevier with Robert Sevier

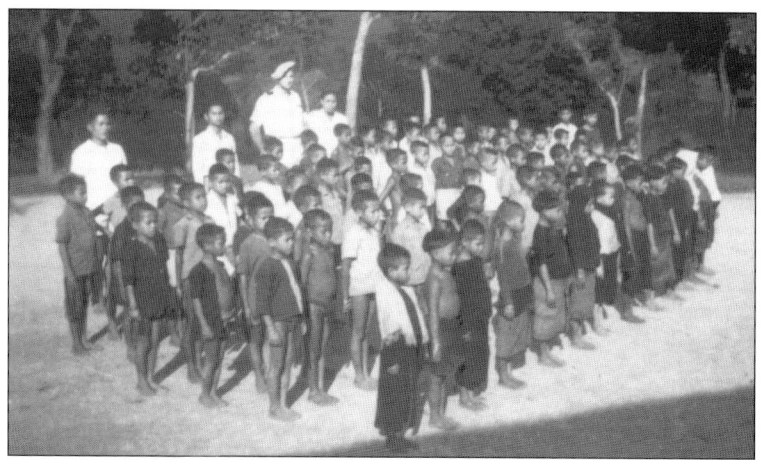

Montagnard children

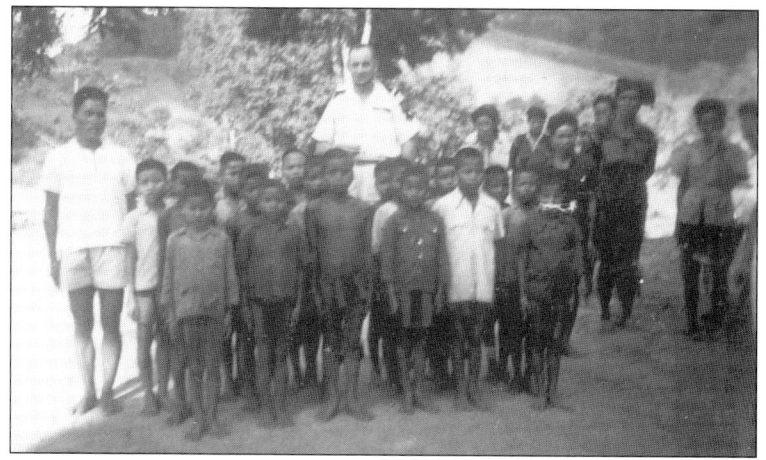

School

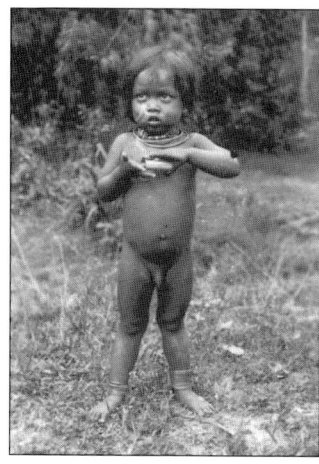

Montagnard child with beriberi

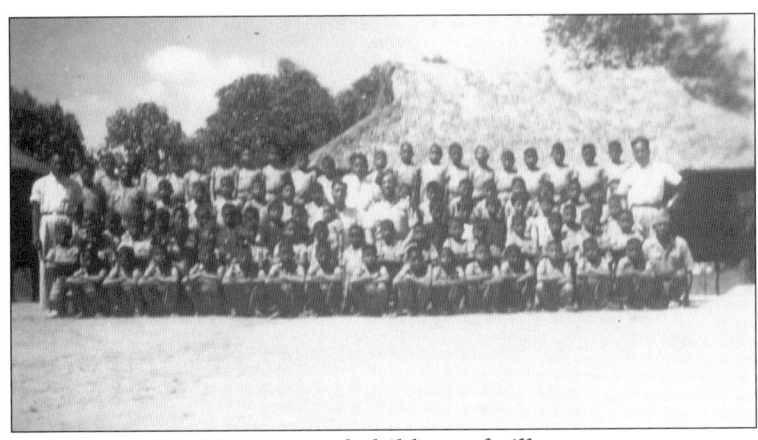
Montagnard children of village

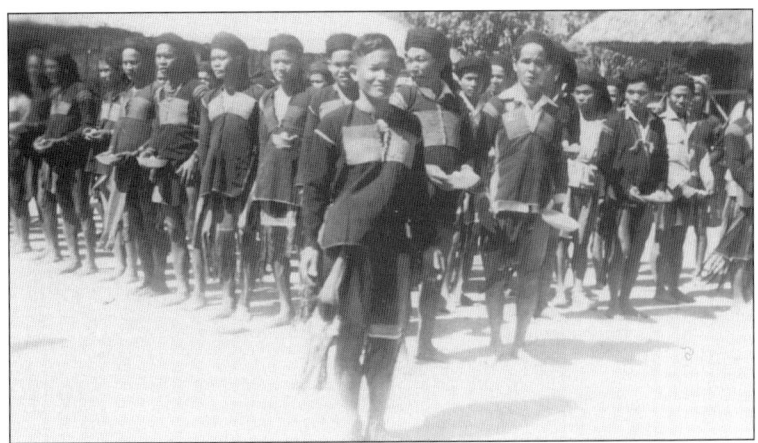
Montagnards at village

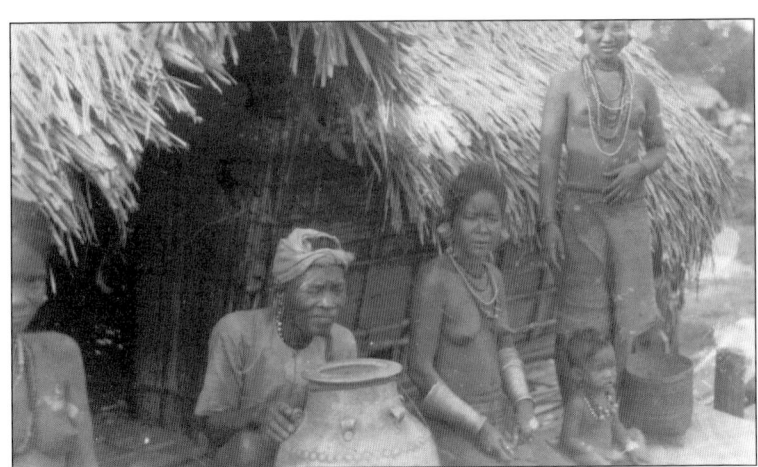
Village M' Drack

War Without a Front

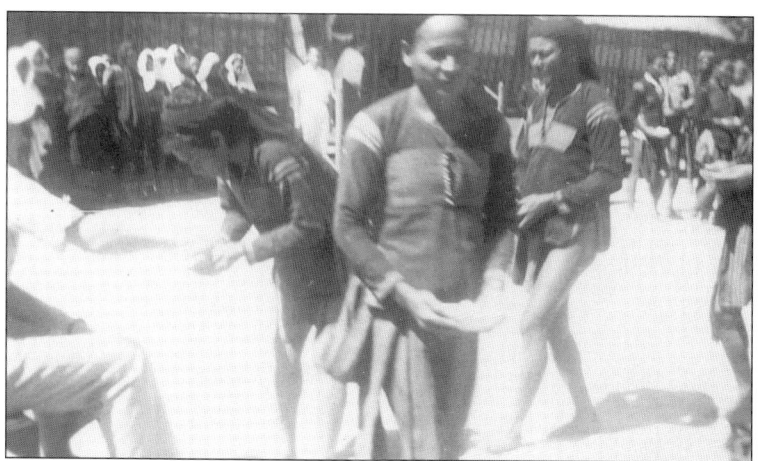

Children honoring Philippe

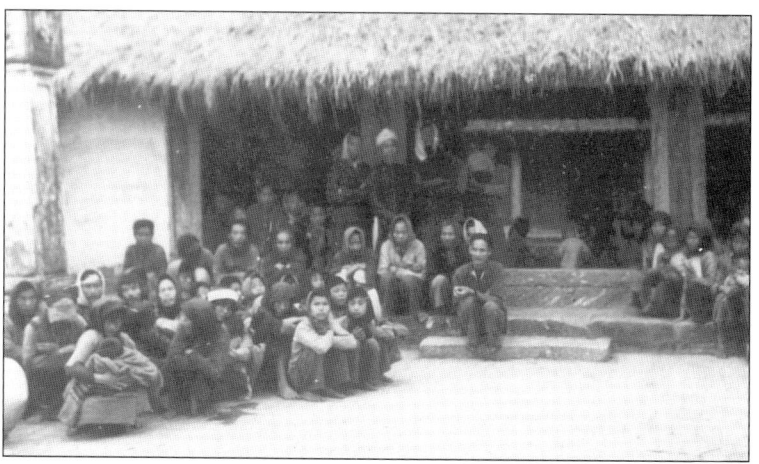

Montagnard school

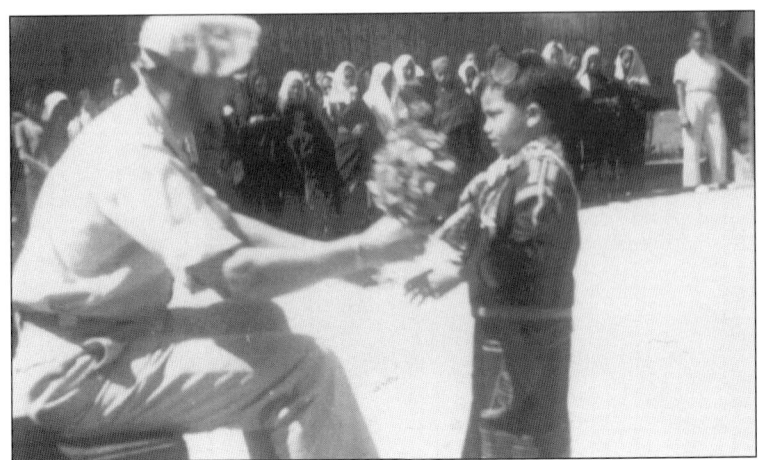

Philippe teaching child

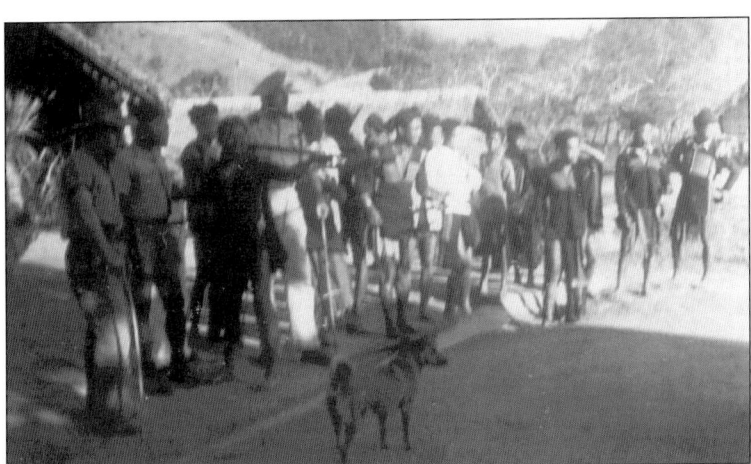

Philippe teaching Montagnards to shoot

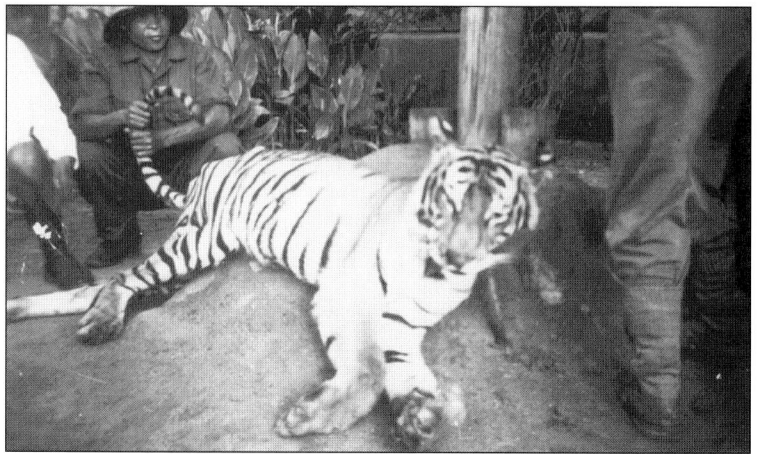

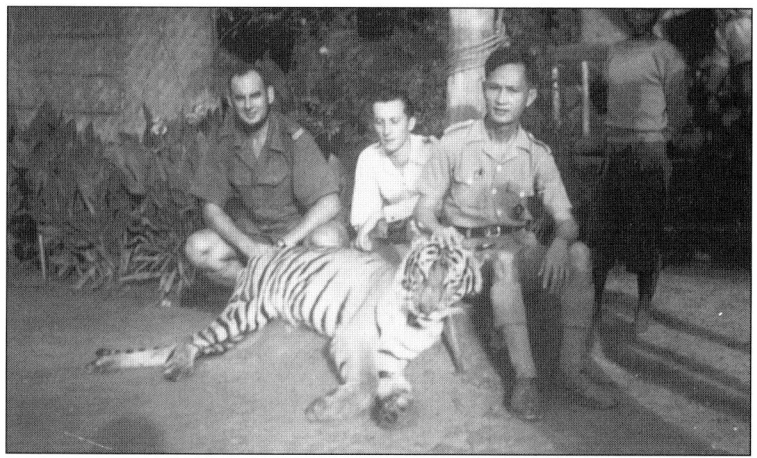

Philippe's tiger

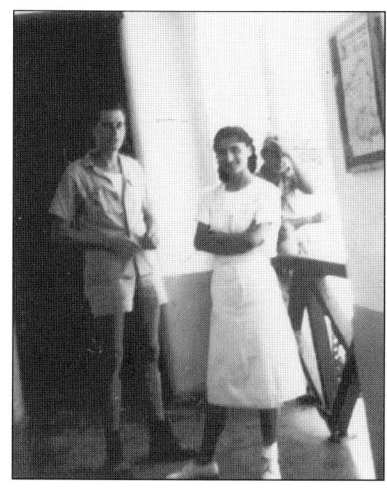

Elisabeth and paramedic

Elisabeth Sevier with Robert Sevier

Chapter 9
Viet Minh Buildup

*U*pon returning to work after my Da Lat vacation, I discovered that the Viet Minh had increased their activities around Hue. As a result, the hospital was full of casualties with more coming in each day. During R and R, I had been lulled into a peaceful state, but immediately after returning to the hospital I was shocked back into the reality of the war. As I made my rounds, I kept wondering how much longer it would last and I really questioned its purpose. France had been fighting for so many years (sending troops shortly after the end of World War II) and still had made no real progress toward a peaceful solution. In addition, we were treating increasing numbers of civilian casualties, including old men, women, and children. Seeing small children suffer was a new and particularly difficult experience for me; I had only treated soldiers when in the Resistance.

Late the next afternoon the hospital staff assembled for an unscheduled meeting. Dr. Lariat announced that we had lost one of our new young doctors while he volunteered in the field. While following the patrol, he stepped on a land mine which killed him instantly. I had never even met the new doctor. I could not imagine why he had elected to go on patrol rather than stay in the triage area. The entire staff attended his funeral before he was buried in a Hue military cemetery. Dr. Carlson presided over the services.

The rest of the week passed quickly with the number of wounded increasing each day. We were not staffed adequately to handle the volume, so we worked longer hours just to keep up. The Viet Minh were becoming more aggressive and it seemed their equipment and men had increased dramatically.[17] Many of the wounded complained that the Viet Minh were playing with the French like a cat chases a mouse.

After a week of working both day and night at the hospital, Janine and I were called to set up a triage unit northwest of Quang Tri. We moved out early in the morning with Drs. Mattei, Deit, and Seuzier. Janine and I were the only nurses going along. We arrived at the site at six o'clock the next morning and efficiently set up two operating rooms, a triage area, and a recovery room. The army provided help from the Vietnamese soldiers in the unit. Within two hours, both military and civilian casualties began to arrive. We had more than 20 seriously wounded, including women and children from the village. More than a dozen of our men, as well as uncounted civilians, were killed. It was reported that the Viet Minh had lost many more than the French had, but it did not matter. More Frenchmen were dead and the murder of innocent civilians made the tragedy that much more terrible.

Janine and I worked most of the day and night, taking only a one-hour nap before returning to triage. We were short of blood plasma, but our American advisor flew into Hue and obtained more for our unit. We could not send our casualties out by ambulance because the Viet Minh had taken over the main road around Quang Tri. We could send back only the more seriously wounded, who were flown out by two small airplanes.

Overall, the fighting lasted more than a week. At last, the Viet Minh were pushed back into their usual jungle hiding places. The roads were opened and we transported the remainder of our wounded to Hue by ambulance or truck. It took more than three days to move all the casualties out and pack up our tents and equipment. On July 2, 1952, we arrived back in Hue totally exhausted. I went directly home and slept for more than 19 hours. The next morning, I arrived at the hospital 15 minutes late, the first time I had been tardy since being assigned to the hospital.

Dr. Lariat told me that Philippe had come to see me after I had gone home and would be in Hue until the following day. I was very happy to see Philippe again. We had developed a real bond, the kind that many people never experience. Dr. Lariat had invited Philippe to dine with all of us at the Officers' Club. Over dinner, Dr. Lariat questioned Philippe extensively about his duties with the Montagnards, trying to discern Philippe's view on the progress of the war. Philippe confirmed that the Viet Minh were getting much stronger and more daring in their attacks on the French and loyal Vietnamese forces.

Philippe told us he was going into the mountains during his short vacation to hunt tigers with four Montagnards. Philippe loved to hunt and did so at every opportunity, so the next morning when Janine and I met with him at breakfast he was in an exceptionally good mood. He told me he would give me a tiger skin if he was lucky enough to kill two or more. The first tiger pelt had already been promised to his parents.

On July 5, Dr. Lariat reported that along with Drs. Boof and Mattei, Janine and I were to support OPERATION QUADRILLE. At three o'clock the next morning, we rolled out of the compound and arrived six hours later. By evening we were ready to take casualties and the next morning at 7 o'clock they started to arrive.

Because we did not have enough personnel, the paramedics took over the triage duties and Janine and I worked in surgery with the doctors. The wounded were extremely serious, and included an abnormal amount of chest, leg, and arm injuries caused by mines. The doctors performed the operations and Janine and I closed the wounds. We were fortunate to have three airplanes to transfer our most critical patients to Tourane and Hue. We worked throughout the day and most of the night. Finally, early the next morning, we had a respite and we all were able to sleep about three hours before more incoming wounded arrived. All day we experienced the same horror as yesterday with many men losing their arms and legs. After midnight, as if someone had turned off a faucet, the flow of patients almost ceased. The paramedics told us that the Viet Minh had retreated and we had been successful. *How could we feel any elation over a success that caused so much suffering among our own forces?* We wearily packed up our gear and returned to Hue.

After sleeping for 20 hours, I returned to the hospital and found they had expanded into another building modified to provide more patient beds. I also learned of more tragic news: Cap St. Jacques had been overrun by the Viet Minh. All our personnel had been either killed or captured. The Viet Minh had massacred all of the wounded and sick. I immediately grasped that I had been lucky to have left. I also thought about my daughter buried at the Cap St. Jacques cemetery. I hoped her grave had not been disturbed.

The rest of the week was fairly calm, but we were busy. We gradually cut our patient load by transferring men to the large hospital in Saigon. The more seriously injured were sent home to France by hospital ship.

Our hiatus from action only lasted a short time because the Viet Minh attacked a small town just outside Hue. They came into the village seeking recruits during the night, took all the young men, then burned the entire community to the ground. When we arrived, we discovered that the remaining inhabitants had been wounded or beaten by the Viet Minh. Many were screaming in fear and agony. *How could anyone do this to their own countrymen?*

We set up a small triage station and sorted out the more seriously wounded to be immediately transported to the hospital. Then, while Janine and I were tending to those who had been wounded or beaten, the Viet Minh returned in much larger numbers. Our soldiers set up a defensive posture at the edge of the village while the commander called for badly needed reinforcements. The Viet Minh had surrounded us and began artillery and mortar attacks. We continued to work on our patients throughout the barrage, which lasted all night. We wondered what had happened to the reinforcements we had requested. At the end of the first day, we were swamped with more casualties than we could handle, and we were forced to tend only those who were seriously wounded. Also, we were running out of plasma, bandages, and morphine. Early the next morning, we saw the first French troops arriving in the village. Another French unit was approaching from the opposite side and the Viet Minh were retreating. It was past noon before we could get our ambulances and trucks loaded with the wounded. By five o'clock that evening, the Viet Minh had disappeared into the countryside, but we had treated 100 wounded and pronounced 25 deaths during the siege. Our troops had taken more than 150 prisoners and killed more than 100 during the fight—a slim margin of victory indeed.

At the end of the week we were thrilled to welcome three new nurses to our staff. Juliette was assigned to work and live with Janine and me. She was about our age and specialized in surgical nursing. She was from Toulouse and had reddish blonde hair and beautiful blue eyes. She was bright, animated, and upbeat. We instantly liked one another. The other two nurses were assigned to hospital wards.

The next two weeks were calm, giving us time to tend the wounded and to mend our own bodies and minds. The doctors had some happy news when it was announced that Dr. Boof was promoted to major and Dr. Seuzier to captain. We now had seven doctors and six nurses and we hoped that with the increased staff, field duty could be limited to two weeks at a time.

Janine, Juliette, and I had become such good friends that everyone referred to us as "The Three Musketeers." We were having a good time visiting Hue, touring all the restaurants, and spending quite a bit of time with the Carlsons. We also practiced the Vietnamese language with each other, with special help from our cook and maid. It was a difficult language to speak because subtle pitch differences altered a word's meaning. Consequently, our pronunciation was not good, but we managed to make ourselves understood when we went downtown to the markets and shops.

In the second week of August, Dr. Lariat received word that Drs. Boof, Mattei, and Seuzier plus Janine, Juliette, and myself would replace a crew in a central Vietnam triage station. We were to meet a convoy on the road and continue with them to the camp, but we did not know exactly where we were going. (For security, we no longer received directives that stated precise information concerning our destinations.) After two days on the road we set up a triage station, including cots for us to sleep in when we had time. The soldiers had completed the lookout tower nearby so we felt safe for the moment. We all sat down together and cooked C rations on an open fire (C rations tasted much better when heated).

Immediately after dinner (we did not even get through one game of cards), the artillery fire began. Within the hour, more than 40 wounded and 14 dead were brought into our station. We turned over triage duties to the paramedics and began operating. We had two operating rooms in one large tent and another in a smaller tent. Thank goodness, we had sufficient supplies of plasma, morphine, and medications. I worked with Dr. Mattei and our first patient had to have both legs amputated. After we completed the operations, we immediately air evacuated him to the nearest hospital. The next three patients had taken bullets in the chest. The exit wounds were so large I was surprised that their lungs and hearts had not been destroyed. We worked for more than 24 hours before we had a break. Dr. Mattei and I just fell into our cots and grabbed two hours sleep before returning to duty. Dr. Boof had decided to use two operating rooms and to rotate the other personnel so we could get some rest and be able to function properly.

The next day, we attended to more than 70 wounded. Each team was working for eight hours before being relieved for four hours. The paramedics were helping us clean up and sterilize instruments between operations. We had three sets of instruments so we could keep one set sterilizing in the autoclave at all times. Late that evening, we received a package, by air, from the Carlsons. They had sent cookies, toothbrushes, and toothpaste. They were very welcome and we passed them around as far as they would go.

We were at the station for two weeks with a break of only two days. With one day evolving into the another, I lost track of time. My mind was swimming in thoughts of loss. Our young men were dying and wounded, losing their limbs, and for what purpose? At least, during World War II, we had worked toward a definite goal: defeating Hitler and liberating France. Our mission in Vietnam did not seem to have an objective. Even worse, the French government did not have the determination to provide the needed resources to win the Indochina war, whereas the Viet Minh were gaining strength and resolve as each day passed. I could only pray for peace, something I had not seen for many years.

Haunted by death, I thought of my little Michelle and prayed that she was happy with God. A great feeling of lassitude crept over me.

While in the field, we had not bathed. We only had time to sponge ourselves before going back to work. So when we were relieved by another crew from Tourane and flown back to Hue, I took the time to shower before collapsing for three days.

My tour of duty was coming to an end. I would be free to return home. I could get away from the heat, the blood, and the smell of death. Though it was too late to protect Suzanne from her jerk of a husband, I could be there for her and Maman. Maybe I could even go to America. However, shortly after returning to the hospital from my last field operation, Dr. Lariat asked me to stay in Vietnam an additional six months: "I need experienced people like you to teach the incoming replacements." I knew how desperately nurses were needed and though I was discouraged about the slaughter, I was in decent emotional health. *How could I leave, knowing the staff was desperately shorthanded, and return to a country where no one cared about what I had seen in Indochina?* His request solidified the I thoughts I had harbored about staying: I volunteered for another half year.

Within the next week, we were told about OPERATION CAIMAN, planned to eliminate the Viet Minh forces in central Vietnam. It was hard to return to the area because my only memories of the site were the large number of wounded and dead we had seen two weeks before. We relieved the crew that had replaced us and began getting ready for whatever would come. With Dr. Lariat added to the team, we could set up three operating rooms. Dr. Seuzier was in charge of triage and received help from several paramedics.

Within two hours after setting up triage, we received incoming wounded. My first patient had one-half his head blown off. All we could do was administer massive doses of morphine to stop his pain. He died within an hour. During the first week, we performed numerous amputations which made me physically sick. I remembered how I was in a Paris hospital and told my legs might have to be amputated. Also we lost many patients because of chest wounds. I was amazed that not one of our patients complained.

I felt like I was on a treadmill, walking for days but getting nowhere. I slept and rested when possible, which was not often. By the end of the week, we were all like zombies. Like last time in central Vietnam, we saw so many patients we had stopped counting, but the weather was good and we could promptly airlift our more serious patients to hospitals in Hue and Tourane.

Finally, we had one and one-half days when the fighting decreased and our patient load became minimal. We utilized this time to rest as much as possible. On September 5, 1952, OPERATION CAIMAN ended. Overall, it was estimated that the Viet Minh had suffered 747 casualties and 3,000 were taken as prisoners. It was not announced how many French soldiers were killed and wounded. We packed up and returned to Hue.

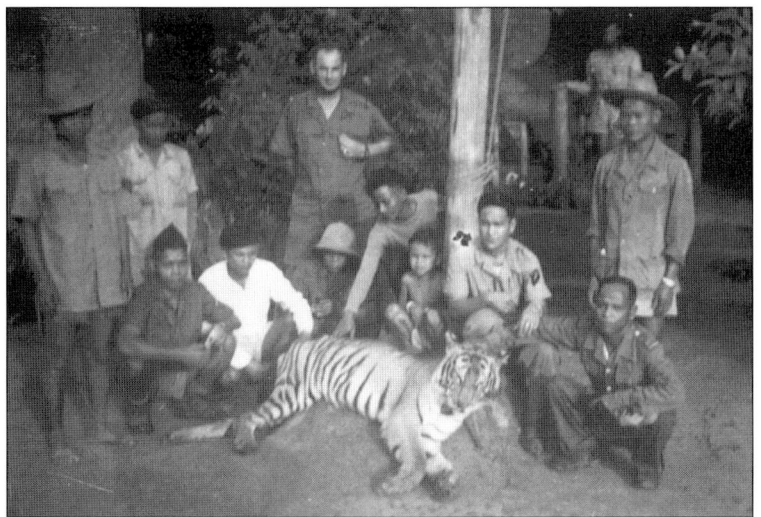

Philippe's Tiger

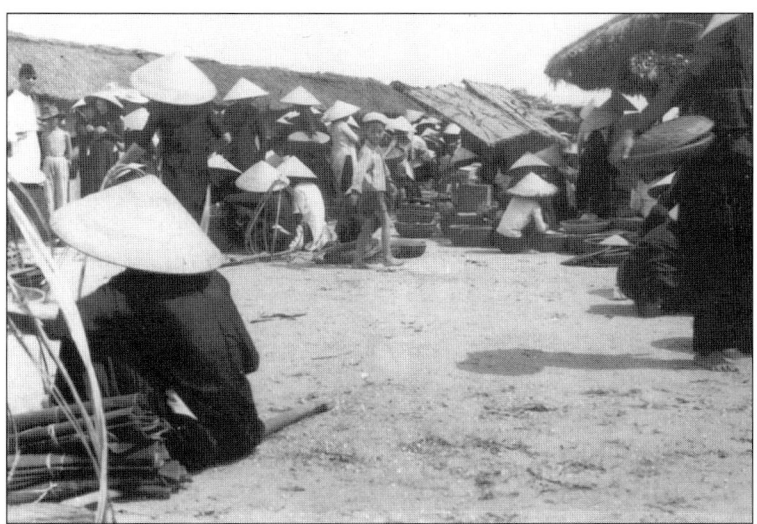

Village near Hue

Chapter 10
War Comes Closer

We resumed our duties at the Hue hospital and for about two weeks, wounded from the battle in central Vietnam kept us quite busy. Then we stabilized and sent most of our patients to Saigon where they were transferred back to France by hospital ship.

Janine, Juliette, and I really appreciated the relatively quiet period. We had time to rest and to visit and read to our patients. The talks always turned to home and family as they eagerly discussed their plans for the future. They never spoke of their time in Vietnam; it was if they had already blocked the memory of the war from their minds. The chaplain was always available, but most preferred to speak to us for some reason. Many had lifetime disabilities and would carry the scars of Vietnam with them forever. They worried constantly about how their loved ones would react to their disabilities. Would they be accepted and could they manage to overcome the loss of a leg or an arm or both? We managed to speak positively and assure them that they would be loved as much as ever.

One of the most discouraging factors in their recovery was the slow mail delivery in Vietnam. A letter from home would do more for their morale than all the medicine we could give them, but most had not received any correspondence in weeks. I always kept a few pictures of my family with me so I could show them. This gave them an excuse to bring out pictures of their families which they usually carried in their wallets. Some of them had young children whom they had never seen because they had been born after their fathers' departure from France to Vietnam. Somehow, just talking to them also raised my own morale. If these brave men could handle the adversities shoved upon them, then my own problems seemed minute. My prayers for their full recovery and future happiness were spoken every night before I retired.

At the end of September 1952, Dr. Lariat informed us that the Viet Minh had attacked three larger villages just outside Hue on the road to Tourane. We set up our team and left early that morning for the area. We arrived within an hour and found nothing left. The villages had been burned to the ground and the only people remaining were on the side of the road. We set up our medical station and began treating all the people who had been lucky enough to make it out of the massacre. Most of the men had been killed or taken by the Viet Minh. The number of small children who were killed and mutilated made us all physically sick. *Why would anyone mutilate a child? To advance a political agenda?* It was too horrible to understand. Hitler may have seemed more systematic, but the Viet Minh were every bit as cruel and calculating as the Nazis.

We spent two weeks at the station taking care of the wounded. The Red Cross from Saigon came and helped us furnish food and reconstruct village huts. The French government set up refugee centers where the Vietnamese could live and eat while rebuilding their villages. Tragically, many of the children had beriberi and their overall degenerative condition made them unable to fight infection and many died. My heart broke as young children, laying gravely ill, looked up at me and smiled. It was particularly horrible when I could only watch as they died from their wounds. Fortunately, we were able to save many of the children, but every child lost became an indelible and profound part of my

Indochinese memories. When our two week rotation ended, I was depressed and felt that death would accompany me forever.

We returned the next day to our duties in the Hue hospital where Dr. Lariat immediately called a briefing of the entire staff. He warned us to be careful where ever we went and to never go anywhere alone. The Viet Minh were becoming much bolder and it was no longer safe even in Hue. He also informed us that several teams would be visiting the villages each week to administer vitamin B-1 shots to the children and hand out information pamphlets, printed in Vietnamese, that explained how a vitamin B–enriched diet can prevent the disease and its complications. The army provided French armed escorts to get us to the villages and back safely. One of our teams, a young doctor named Devaux and a nurse on loan from Saigon had visited a village 10 kilometers from Hue, but the children were in the field and not available for treatment. The medical team returned that evening to complete their mission. They did not tell anyone they were going back and did not have an armed escort. As they were giving the shots to the children in the village, the Viet Minh attacked and they were taken prisoner. The next day they were found dead, tied to a tree, partially naked, mutilated, with red ants crawling all over them. The paramedics cleaned them and brought their bodies back to Hue where they were buried the next day in a full military ceremony. I did not know either one, but it was as if I had lost my best friend. But, for the grace of God, she could have been me. Janine, Juliette, and I had nightmares almost every night for the next month. *Why were medical personnel killed while they were helping poor civilians? How could even the Viet Minh be so barbaric? Why the mutilation of the bodies?* Though I could not understand how thinking individuals could perpetrate extreme brutality for its psychological effects on the survivors, I realized that it worked: my morale had never been so low.

When we reported back to the hospital, we found a welcomed lull with only a few wounded coming in and no military operations near our area. This gave us time to gather ourselves together and attend to personal affairs. We were able to visit with the Carlsons at least twice a week. Most of the conversation centered around the wonders of the United States, especially its size and majestic scenery. I became more determined to see it for myself.

During the middle of October, the Viet Minh attacked and captured a village right outside Quang Tri. They were using the plundered town as a base to completely surround Quang Tri. Our troops were given the mission of searching out and destroying the enemy troops within the area. They spearheaded two separate operations to break the siege.

We packed up again and headed for an area just behind battalion headquarters. Within an hour of setting up operations, we heard the distant sounds of our artillery and mortars. Shortly thereafter, we received the wounded. They all came at once. According to our patients, the fighting was fierce with the Viet Minh securely entrenched and heavily armed. We had set up three operating rooms and kept all three busy for the next week.

The second morning I heard a voice calling to me but in my fatigue I could not place it. I turned and found Roger, my ex-husband. He was laying on a stretcher in the triage area and was suffering from a chest wound. I went over and spoke to him, trying to comfort him. He was taken into the operating room of Dr. Boof where I had been working. I informed Dr. Boof that I was too close to Roger to even think of helping with the operation. I switched places with Janine and assisted Dr. Mattei. Within three hours, Roger was out of the recovery room. His injury, although serious, was not life threatening and he would be all right. I told Roger that everything was fine and we would be moving him to Saigon as soon as possible. He told me Paula had married someone else: "Now I know I should have stayed with you because I still love you."

I looked squarely in his eyes, "I no longer love you." However, since I had finally accepted that the divorce was in our best interests and no longer harbored guilt over it, I had found forgiveness easier. I was at a fork in the road: I could be hostile or I could be kind. I had seen too much hatred to pick the former. I wanted to remain friends. I asked him to write me after he was repatriated to France and let me know how he was doing. Before he was sent to Saigon three days later, I hugged Roger and told him, "I will always be a friend you can depend on."

After Roger departed, I grew sad knowing that our marriage could have been much different. I also thought about my decision to extend my stay in Vietnam and wondered if I had made the right choice. This mood only lasted a short time and I threw myself back into my work. We were busy for the next week with an ever-continuing stream of patients. One day melted into the next, with the same routine: We worked as long as we could, rested for a few hours, and then went back to work. Fortunately, we had sufficient transportation facilities to move our patients when they were physically capable of traveling. We used air transport for the most seriously wounded and trucks and the train for the others.

After we were relieved by another crew from Tourane, we climbed into trucks and headed back to Hue. Within 15 minutes of the time we left the area, the convoy commander received a message sending us to Dong-Hoi. A band of Viet Minh had been harassing the village and they needed our help. We were there within an hour, set up our medical station, and immediately tended the 10 wounded waiting for treatment. The soldiers told us they had begun a mission with the local Vietnamese troops. Immediately after departing from their base, the Vietnamese soldiers deserted, leaving the patrol at less than one-half strength. This situation was becoming a serious problem as many colonial Vietnamese troops were defecting to the Viet Minh. The patrol was ambushed and all the remaining men had been wounded, primarily by sniper fire. They compared it with being targets in a shooting gallery. Fortunately, a follow-up patrol came to their rescue and they were evacuated to our medical station. We stayed in the area for three days while French reinforcements cleared the area of Viet Minh. We were lucky it was a small ambush and the rest of the time was relatively calm with only a few more wounded coming in for treatment.

I arrived in Hue, happy to back to running water and hot food. I had the next day off which I used to wash clothing, write letters home, and just rest and relax. I returned to work at the hospital, happy to be back in civilization again, and was asked if I would accompany Dr. Mattei to a small village just outside Hue. A young mother had been stricken with typhoid. We treated the mother and her baby before transporting them to our hospital. Then we tried to explain to the rest of the villagers why they should boil their drinking water, but the idea of sterilization was completely foreign to them: "Our parents never boiled the drinking water, so why should we?" They took our pamphlets and listened intensely while we explained, but it was evident that the importance of our message was not getting through to them. Within two weeks, the mother and baby were doing well and I was encouraged: at least we were helping.

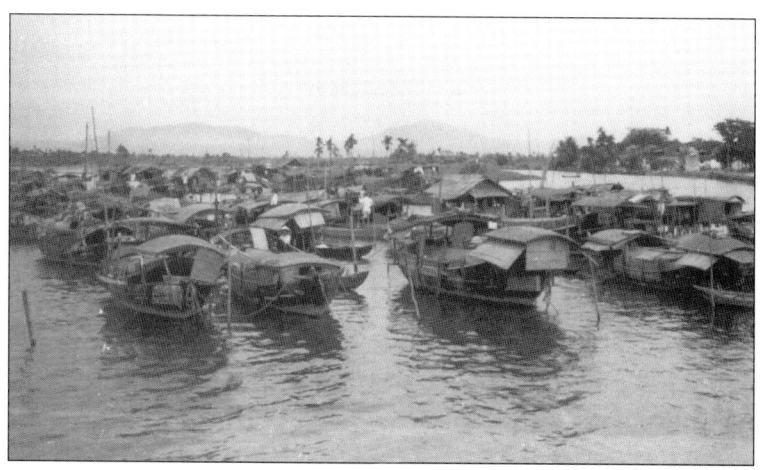

Sampans in Hue

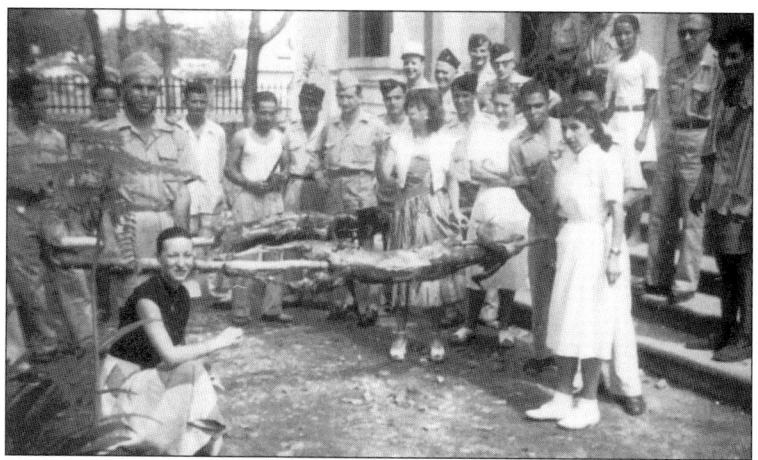

Village children

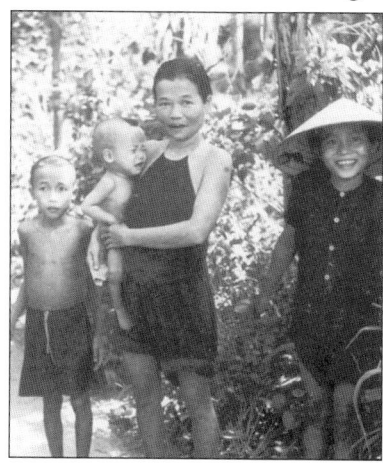

Elisabeth's maid (Hue) and her children

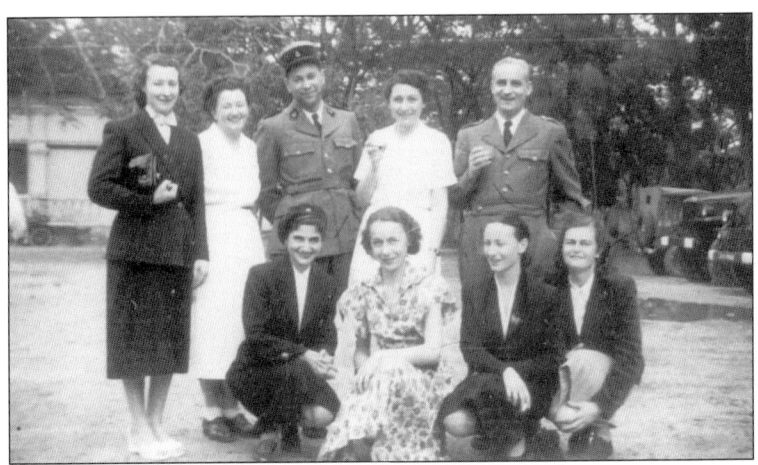

Hue medical team

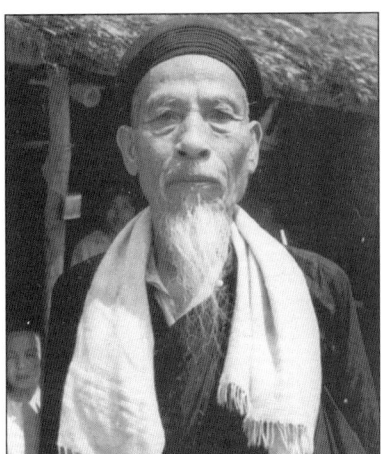

Village chief

Chapter 11
Airborne Training and Return to Laos

During the first week of November 1952, Dr. Lariat asked for volunteers to take airborne training. The Viet Minh had continued to augment their forces in Laos, and our commanders believed the buildup must be checked. An extensive network of jungle trails lead into Vietnam and the Viet Minh were using these footpaths to infiltrate Laos and take over the country. However, there were few roads in Laos and the only quick access to our camps was by parachute. Janine, Juliette, and I immediately applied for jump school as did Drs. Lariat, Boof, and Mattei. We received word within three days from Saigon that we had been selected to attend airborne medical training, where we would learn how to drop into remote French camps and provide services. Fifteen paramedics also had been chosen.

We reported to a paratrooper camp, about 100 kilometers from Hue, near Quang Tri. We were assigned quarters and began training the next morning. The camp was isolated, in the woods and well hidden by surrounding trees, but had full airport facilities.

We were totally exhausted at the end of each day. During the first week, training consisted of four hours of extensive exercise and physical training. In the afternoon we learned how to use a parachute, how to land, and how to pack the chute. The second week began with our first jump. I was the third jumper on the first run. Drs. Lariat and Boof went before me. I got to the door and froze. The jump-master just looked at me, smiled, and gave me a gentle shove out of the plane. The experience took my breath away. It was beautiful outside and I felt as if I was completely free. I was brought to abrupt attention when my parachute opened. It was quite a jolt. I marveled at the sense of floating down. I hit the ground, rolled with my landing as I had been instructed, and gathered the parachute toward me. Then I ran to join the others. I felt such joy! We made four more jumps and I did not need another push! That night we all celebrated; I remember how good the food tasted at camp. I guess the intense physical activity had increased my appetite. We all completed five jumps each day for the rest of the week. At the end of the week, the paratroopers held a ceremony and presented all of us with paratrooper badges and honorary French paratrooper red berets. We also received bonuses for successfully completing the training. On the way back to Hue, we only talked of parachuting; Janine, Juliette, and I were happy we had volunteered for this special training. The doctors and paramedics also seemed very pleased with their experiences.

Within the week, we received word that our unit would be sent to the Laotian Plain of Jars, an elevated plateau in the Xieng Khoung province. The highlands were called the Plain of Jars because huge abandoned urns, the last remainders of a previous unknown civilization, were found there.[18] The elevation was approximately 3,400 feet, the climate mild, and resources rich. Most Laotian cattle were raised in the Plain of Jars and many fruits were grown there.

We packed up and left Hue in a military convoy. After a five-hour jeep journey, we arrived at the Laotian border. In an empty field, we slept overnight in the ambulances. Early the next morning, we received word that the paratroopers operating in a mountain camp had been in a firefight overnight and sustained numerous wounded. Dr. Lariat and the battalion commander sent in a medical team to take care of the situation until further help could arrive. Drs. Lariat, Boof, and Mattei as well as Janine, Juliette, and I, were selected to make the jump. We took off from the airstrip and flew for an hour before we arrived at the site. A French paratrooper unit was already on the ground. I jumped and felt the same feeling of joy and freedom I had experienced during the training jumps. I was looking at the beautiful plains and enjoying every moment when I hit the ground. I forgot to roll as I had been instructed and hurt my left leg. I could not walk so two paratroopers helped me to the camp where Dr. Lariat informed me that my left ankle was sprained. He put a walking cast on my leg and I spent the rest of the time in Laos hobbling. The medical equipment was on site and 15 patients were already waiting for us. We set up three operating rooms, a triage area, and a recovery tent.

A company of seasoned paratroopers had been on patrol and ambushed during the night. Two had been killed and the others were critically wounded. Many of the Officers and Non-Commissioned Officers were veterans of World War II. I worked with Dr. Lariat, Juliette with Dr. Mattei, and Janine with Dr. Boof. Of the 15 men treated, we had lost three before we could operate. Six of the wounded had to undergo amputations, two with an arm, three with one leg, and one poor soldier who needed both legs removed. He had stepped on a mine and there was not enough left of the limbs to save. It was such a heart wrenching experience for all of us. We finally completed work on the last patient late that evening and sat down to eat some heated C-rations. We were all so tired and demoralized; we hardly spoke while eating.

Early the next morning, we were awakened when new patients began coming in. The remainder of our unit had arrived during the night and the paramedics had set up their triage station. During that day and night, we received more than 80 wounded and worked well into the night. We did not have time to breathe between operations. The wounded were still coming in after midnight but the numbers declined and we were able to free up two teams for a short rest. Dr. Lariat also took a break while I completed the suturing with the help of a paramedic. After I finished, I was able to sleep for two hours.

I woke up and the rest of the crew was already working hard. I took time out to visit the recovery tent and talk to some of the patients we had treated the night before. I searched for the double amputee we had treated, but the paramedic on duty told me he had died during the night.

My morning started like that of the prior day: incoming wounded arrived faster than we could treat them. All night long, the operating room tables were occupied. Ten major operations had been performed during the night. The paratroopers' battalion had been surrounded by Viet Minh who used mortars and grenades to inflict heavy casualties. We treated numerous chest and stomach wounds as well as an unusually high number of limb wounds. The recovery tent was filled with agonizing groans and stertorous breathing. The operating rooms sounded with the rustle of moving arms, the murmur of voices, the clink of surgical instruments, and the slash and click of surgical scissors. We were finally able to rest after four o'clock the next morning.

The break lasted only four hours when the injured began coming in. During the week, we operated on more than 250 patients, averaging only about three hours rest each day. We lost more patients than I had ever experienced before. Our paratroopers informed us that the Viet Minh had modern weapons and their numbers were very large. Our troops were making progress in stabilizing the area but the cost was heavy.

The second week began as the first had ended. Each day brought us more and more wounded. We worked more than 36 hours during one period. We were working on instinct and adrenaline. The carnage was so great and I was so fatigued that my memory became blurred. However, one moment I shall never forget. After we had amputated a leg from a very large soldier, I asked one of the paramedics to help me take the leg to a small tent where we stored amputated limbs. When he opened the tent, I was stunned and horrified by the innumerable bloody and bare arms and legs stacked inside tent. I hastily turned away, went to my tent, drank some water, and swallowed two aspirins. The paramedics and orderlies soon buried the arms and legs, but I could not erase the image from my mind. Even now, years later, I can recall with vivid clarity that huge stack of severed limbs and the tragic look of our patients when they awoke from surgery and discovered an arm or leg missing.

The paratroopers drove back the Viet Minh during the second week and secured the primary trails that the enemy had been using to move supplies from Laos into Vietnam. We left after 15 days and returned to Hue.

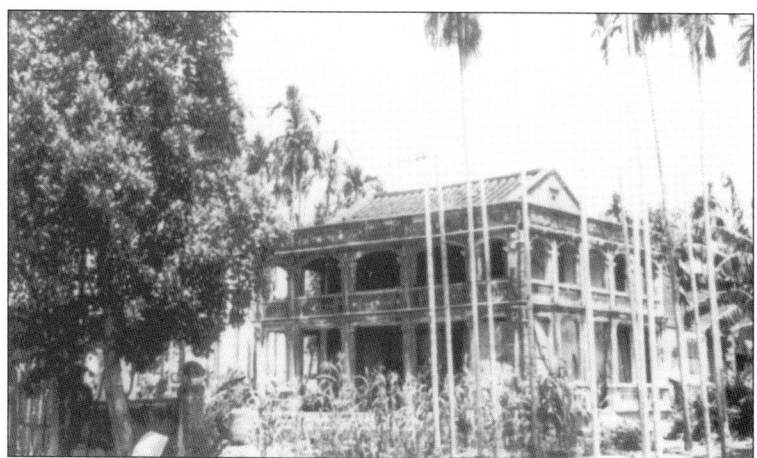
Laotian residence

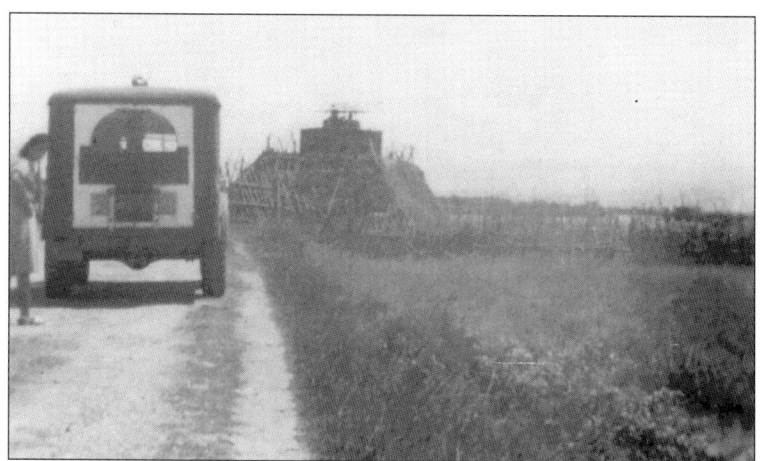
Rest stop on way to Laos

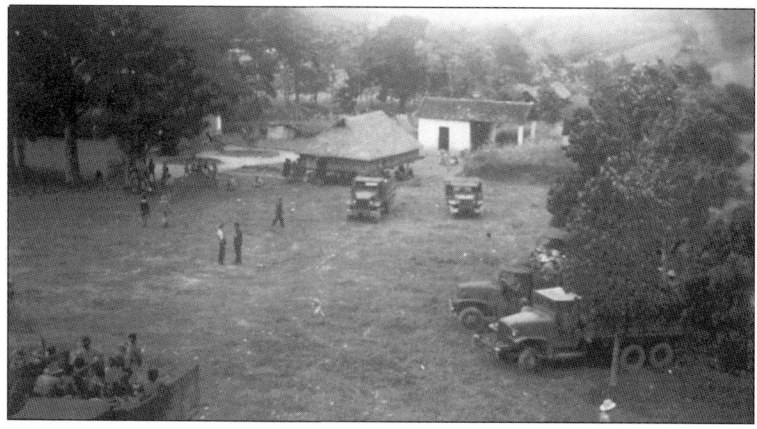
French Camp — Laos

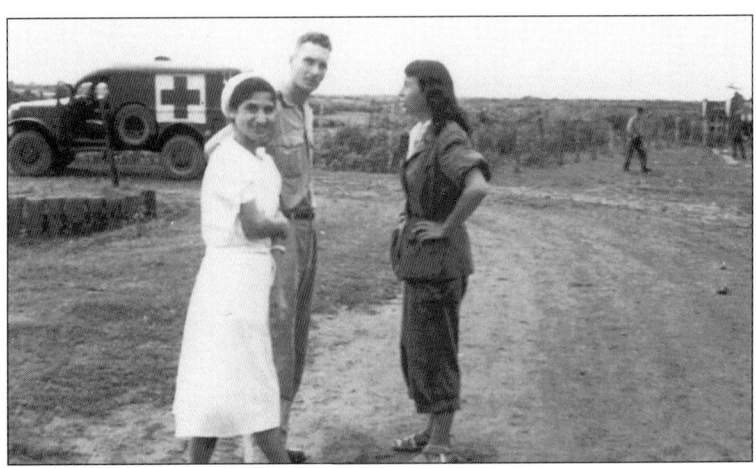

On the road to Laos

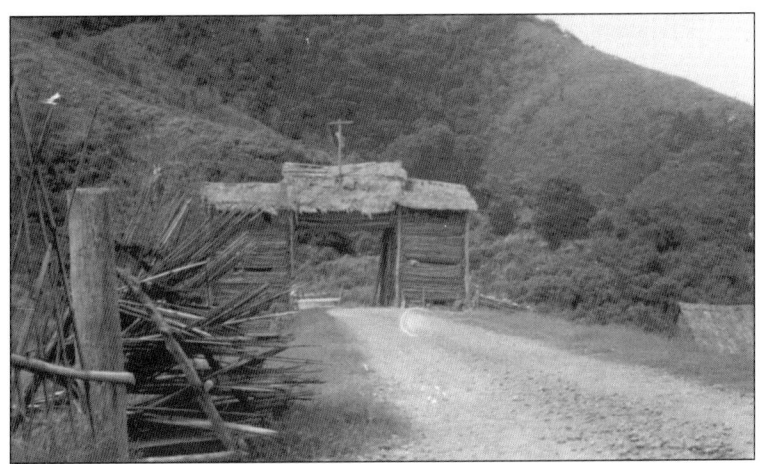

On the road to Laos

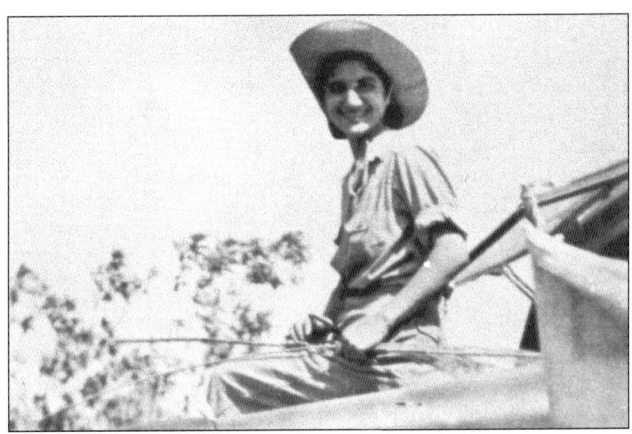

Elisabeth

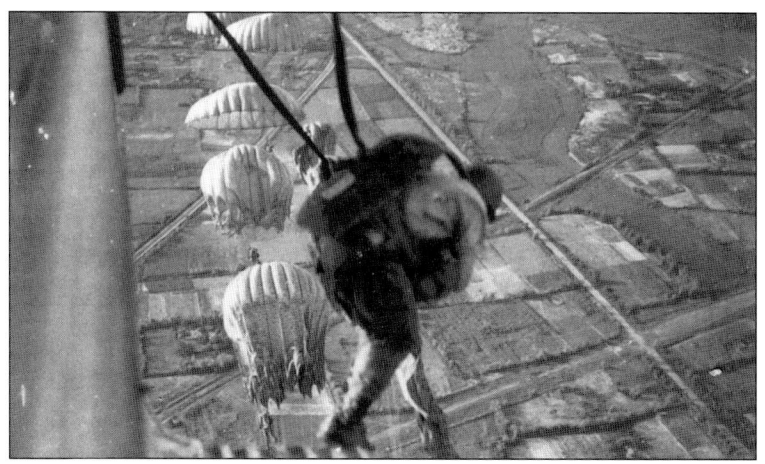

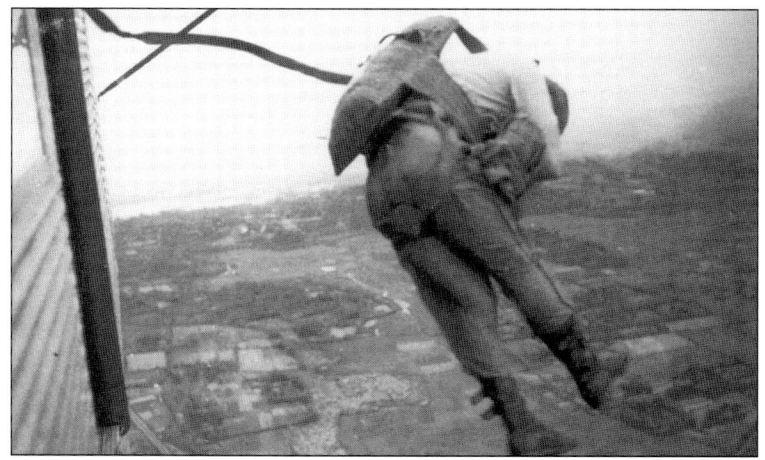

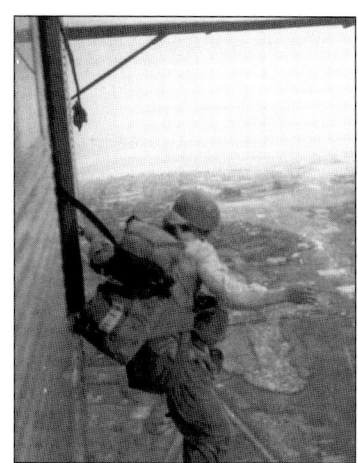
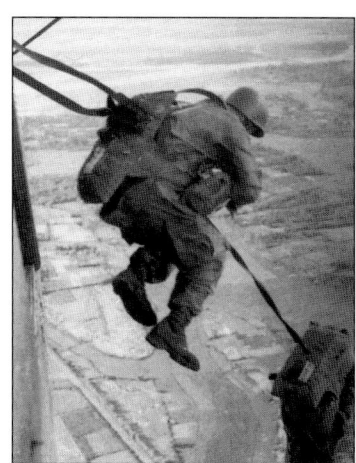

Airborne training

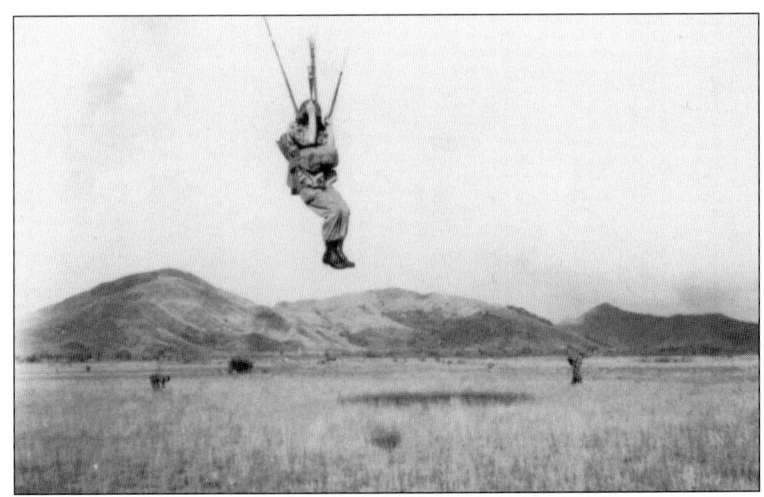

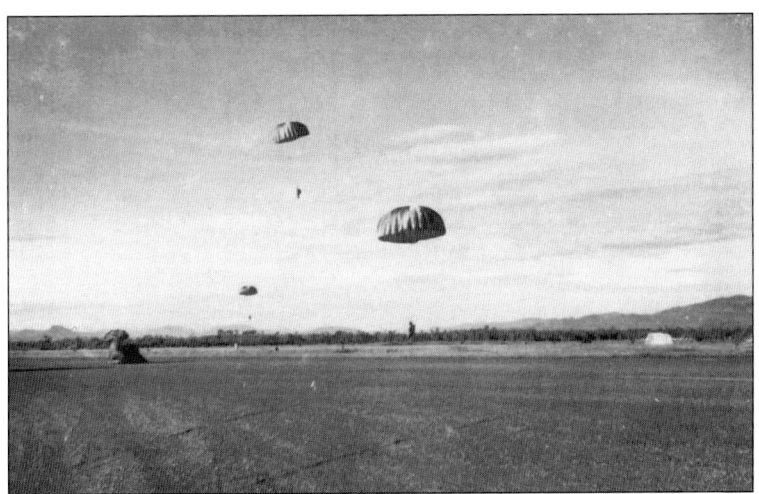

Parachute training

Chapter 12
Nam Dinh and the End of the Tour

When we arrived in Hue, we were all given five days off. We were all exhausted and demoralized from the experience in Laos. Most of the time was used for rest and sorting out our feelings. The Carlsons came over to the house and helped us overcome our depression.

When I returned to work after the short vacation, the hospital was still full of patients from the fighting in Laos and nearby skirmishes. I grew especially fond of a young paratrooper who had both legs amputated. I stopped by his bed at every opportunity to visit with him and read him old newspapers. He was only 21 years old and had been in the army since graduating from high school. Named Christophe, he had dark hair and dark brown eyes and had been in Indochina about a year. It was heartbreaking to see so much sadness in the eyes of such a fine young man. He had been one of my patients in Laos and always greeted me with a large smile and some kind of kidding remark. He wished desperately to return to his home in Marseilles to see his parents before dying. He had developed gangrene and his prognosis was poor. I spent as much time as possible with him, and when he asked me to write to his mother because he was too weak to hold the pen, I was happy to oblige. As each day passed, he became worse and finally he died while I was at his side. Janine had also spent a lot of time with him and we both cried and prayed for him. He had never complained and held a positive attitude until the moment he died. His death was nothing but a waste. Janine and I both wrote a letter to his mother telling her how bravely he had died and how much he had wanted to go home and see his family. We assured her that he was not alone when he died and that we cared for him very much.

We were in the hospital another two weeks before it was announced that OPERATIONS BRETAGNE, ARTOIS, and NORMANDIE would be launched southwest of Nam Dinh, approximately 50 kilometers south of Hanoi, where the Viet Minh had more than 15 battalions in place. These would be the largest operations to date in Indochina, designed to destroy the Viet Minh bases once and for all. Four doctors and five nurses from Tourane, and three doctors and three nurses (Janine, Juliette, and I) from Hue headed to Nam Dinh.

On December 20, 1952, we left with five ambulances and 15 paramedics, escorted by a battalion of paratroopers. As we drove along the road, we observed a large group of Vietnamese civilians who were being evacuated for their safety by the French. They were carrying the few possessions they could take with them on their backs and on their wagons and bicycles. The scene reminded me of the flight of Parisians during World War II. It was obvious from their looks and gestures that they considered the French responsible for their homelessness.

The battle began early on Christmas Eve, two days after we arrived, and by late afternoon, we received our first wounded. We worked constantly until after midnight. It was cold in our tent and the dull ache in my legs and back hampered my effectiveness. When we finally finished, we had treated more than 100 wounded and we could tell it was a large military operation. I managed to get three hours sleep and a cup of coffee before reporting back to our operating tent.

My legs and back were hurting me so much that I could hardly walk. I attributed my discomfort to fatigue and reasoned that I had probably contracted a cold. We attended more wounded during the day, although not nearly as many as the previous evening. When I went back to my tent that night, I was shivering. I wrapped myself in blankets and tried to sleep. I managed four hours rest before waking with a terrible headache. My legs and back seemed to be worse, which prompted Dr. Lariat to give me a pain pill. I managed to work the rest of the day, but moved so slowly I contributed very little. Janine took my temperature which was higher than normal. Dr. Lariat gave me some quinine and informed me that I had an attack of malaria or influenza.[19] The weather remained cold and Dr. Lariat told me to sleep in the ambulance, but I had trouble resting there and did not want to be alone. I moved into the tent and Dr. Lariat took my temperature, which had risen to 102 degrees. I woke up the next morning feeling weak and with a throbbing headache, but I was able to eat some hot soup and managed to help in the triage area for two hours. However, later in the day, I was in so much pain I had to go back to my tent and lay down. Dr. Lariat sent Janine to stay with me. She was worried about me and I felt very lucky to have such a good friend.

The next day, Dr. Mattei told me I was going to be evacuated back to the hospital in Hue. I tried to convince him that I could recover without being moved, but he was insistent, and on December 27, 1952, I was flown out of Nam Dinh. I arrived at the hospital and was placed in a small isolation room with a very high window. I was not at all happy about returning, but I was not getting any better and seemed to be losing strength each day. Sometime during the night, I began hallucinating. I saw lots of flowers but every time I would reach for them; their location would change. My fever increased to 103 degrees and the doctor assigned a Vietnamese nurse to stay with me throughout the night. Dr. Giraud, who was new to the hospital, took blood to be sent to Saigon for analysis. The next few days passed with my temperature dropping to 101 degrees. The blood test came back within 24 hours and showed that I had paratyphoid, which was probably caused by an inoculation I had taken two months before. Since I did not have infectious typhus, Dr. and Mrs. Carlson were allowed to visit me. They had come to my room every day even when I was quarantined and unable to receive visitors.

I improved the next few days and was looking forward to being discharged. Unfortunately, I took a turn for the worse. My temperature soared and I began sweating profusely. During the night, my fever became so high that the nurses gave me cold sponge baths every two to three hours and I perspired so much they had to change my sheets every few hours. Mrs. Carlson came and spent most of the day with me. She was always optimistic and her pleasant demeanor helped my morale. She would hug me and tell me I would soon be well and out of the hospital; however, I did not get well and one morning I did not even have the strength to turn myself. I was sleeping most of the time under heavy morphine sedation and in and out of a delirium that was punctuated with hallucinations. I saw three figures, all with my face, who were laughing at me. I would close my eyes to rid myself of these images, but could not sleep or rest soundly.

One early morning, when the nurse was attending me, I asked her to feel my face to ensure that I was still alive. She took my temperature which remained above 103 degrees. That evening she brought me some brandy and I drank it. I slept soundly all night for the first time in over a week. The following morning my fever had completely subsided. I had lost most of my hair and my weight was down to 70 pounds, but I continued to make a little progress each day. My mind began to function normally as I began to think of my friends and work again. My unit was still in the field and I welcomed all the news from them each day.

My unit came back from the battle near Nam Dinh early the next week. I was ecstatic to see them. They had become my family. Dr. Lariat came by each day as did most of the others. Janine and Juliette pampered me like I had never been treated before. They took turns sitting with me every night until I went to sleep. We talked about everything, good times and bad. We had been through so much together, we even thought the same way. They had become sisters in spirit to me. The Carlsons also came by each day and we talked about my impending departure from Vietnam. They told me how much they hoped I would someday go to America and see the wonders they had talked about and shown through their wonderful color slides.

In mid-January 1953, I was still bedridden and the Hue area was under intense attack from the Viet Minh. I could hear the sounds of distant artillery every night. I desperately wanted to be able to get up, to be able to help my fellow workers who were exceptionally busy; I was depressed because I had to lie around when there was so much work to be done. As a result, I grew short and irritable with my nurse. She finally said, "Grow up. You're very lucky to be alive." However, I did not want to accept my physical limitations. I was determined to get out of bed. One night, I tried to get up while the others were sleeping. Slowly, I climbed out of bed and tried to stand up, but my legs were too weak and I fell back into my bed. Determined to stand, I immediately tried again. I was able to stand on my feet near my bed for a few minutes and it felt wonderful. I worked on building my leg strength each day and began taking short walks. By the next week, I was able to dress myself and make it to the bathroom on my own.

It felt good to be independent again, but when I looked in the mirror, I did not recognize myself. I looked like a skeleton, and the little hair I still had came out in large hunks whenever I tried to comb it. Dr. Lariat, while pleased with my progress, told me that my head needed to be shaved because I would soon lose all of my hair anyway. "Don't worry Elisabeth, it will grow back thicker than before." The next day, Janine and Juliette came into my room with a gift wrapped up in a large festive box. Inside was a wig that they had bought in a local beauty shop. The hair was long, down past my shoulders, and very black. I put it on and they laughed, "You've gone native! If you had any color in your face, you'd look Vietnamese."

During the first week of February, I received my orders to return to France. I was both sad and happy about leaving. I had seen enough tragedy and death to last a lifetime but I had also molded wonderful relationships with the nurses, doctors, and paramedics. I would really miss Janine, Juliette, and Drs. Lariat, Boof, and Mattei. (Dr. Lariat received his orders to return home before I left and departed by air immediately for a month's vacation in La Martinique.)

I flew from Hue to Tourane where I completed some paperwork and then flew onto Saigon. I stayed in the hospital for a week and I went back to Cap St. Jacques and visited the grave of my Michelle. I bought a large bouquet of flowers and placed it on her grave. I spent the day with her at the cemetery before flying back to Saigon that night. I departed the next morning, February 25, on the *S.S. Kerquelen*.

My top-deck cabin had a bed, a small refrigerator with a mini-bar, and a bathroom and shower. I met two other nurses who were also returning home and they lifted my spirits. Sarah was happy and vivacious and Angele more reserved. We quickly became friends. They had worked as staff nurses for a year in Saigon.

I was assigned to work in the ship's hospital to help attend the 200 wounded patients on-board, primarily to give the regular ship nurses a break. Since I only worked 3–6 hours daily, I had sufficient time off to relax and enjoy the sun. I ate in the Officers' Mess on board and the food was delicious. I also used the library and lounge to occupy my spare time. The sea was calm and the waves striking the hull of the boat had a lulling effect on me. The nights were beautiful with the moon beaming down onto the ship and the sea. I was enjoying my first trip on a large boat. The serenity of the voyage compared to my frantic days in Vietnam was just what I needed. I loved to stand on the deck and watch the waves and reflect on my experiences in Indochina while the big vessel pushed forward.

Sarah, Angele, and I toured Singapore where we docked for two days. We visited the city market and shopped. In the streets, we could hear almost every language: French, German, Chinese, English, and various others. It was so hot and humid we could not stay outside very long, so after lunch we returned to the ship which had air conditioning. The next day, the ship's captain arranged a tour of the city. Fifteen passengers were loaded on a small bus and a French-speaking, Indian tour guide told us about the Natural Museum, the Raffles Hotel, and the Botanical Gardens. The tour lasted most of the day and we arrived back at the ship late in the afternoon, hot and tired. We had dinner on the ship and then went directly to bed. I was so tired that I slept until noon the next day.

The sea remained calm but the weather began to get much hotter as we approached the equator. The captain warned us not to spend too much time in the sun because of its intensity. Sarah, Angele, and I went out on the deck chairs to sun early in the morning. We went inside for lunch and then made the mistake of returning to the deck for more sun. Angele left about two hours later, but Sarah and I had fallen asleep and did not wake up until five o'clock in the afternoon. When I got to my room, I felt dizzy and so tired that I fell asleep. When I woke up 12 hours later, I had a high fever, was sick to my stomach, and had a splitting headache. I got up from bed and immediately threw up. I had heat stroke. The doctor prescribed an IV with normal saline and instructed me to drink as much water as possible. He had a nurse look in on me during the rest of the night and the next day.

My body and head were as red as fire and my skin was horribly burned. The doctor gave me pain medication and had the nurse apply balm to ease my pain, but I still remained in bed for three days. When I was able to get up and navigate, I had to move very slowly because any movement of clothing against my blistered skin was excruciating. My sunning days were over!

Within a week, when we were between Singapore and Colombo, I was all right, but a lot wiser. When the captain announced over the intercom that we had crossed the equator, we all assembled on the deck to celebrate. We had been issued special sunglasses to use when viewing the sun, which looked orange and close enough to touch. It was a beautiful sight and so quiet I could hear the small waves brushing across the bow of the ship. Never before had I felt closer to the beautiful universe that God had created.

We arrived in Colombo a few days later where we stayed for two days. Colombo was the capital seaport of Ceylon (now Sri Lanka). The ship's officers advised us to visit the Walfendahl Church built in 1749. Sarah, Angele, and I took a cab to the beautiful church and later we went to the city market and bought some colorful cotton blouses. I bought one for Maman, one for Suzanne, and two for myself. We decided to stop at a small cafe where we ordered the Lanka's tea, which was dark and very tasty. The people were pleasant to us and we ended the evening by going to the harbor and watching the boats go by. One fascinating aspect of Colombo was the variety of languages heard; it seemed as if every nation in the world was represented. However, the charm of Colombo was tainted by the large number of street beggars who stopped everyone as they passed. It was definitely a two-class society representing the very rich and the very poor.

The next day we entered the Gulf of Aden in the Arabian Sea where we sailed for 10 days before entering the Red Sea. Finally, after waiting behind heavy traffic for a over a day, we passed through the Suez Canal. Though we worked only four days a week and were enjoying ourselves, I was anxious to get home.

I was glad that we stopped in Cairo for food and supplies because it gave me an opportunity to see the pyramids. Along with a tour group, I spent two hours touring the Giza Pyramid, then proceeded to the Saqqara Pyramid, which had been erected in 2900 B.C, but I did not have time to go inside of it.

The next day, when we arrived at the Mediterranean Sea, I felt like we were home at last. We arrived in Marseilles on March 23, 1953, where we were greeted with a military band, the mayor, and other dignitaries. We had lunch with the official party on the ship and the mayor presented all the nurses with large bouquets of roses. As the wounded were taken off the ship, the band played "The Marseillaise." I was among the last to debark and was taken to the military hospital in Marseilles. I stayed there three days for a complete physical examination before being granted a 36-day leave.

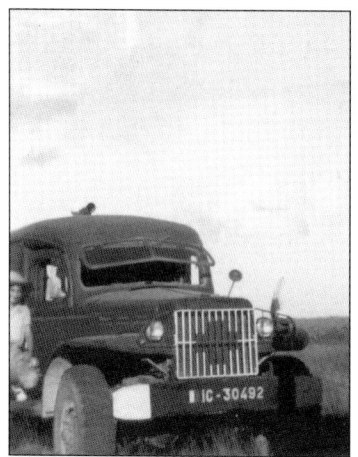
Ambulance at Nam Dinh

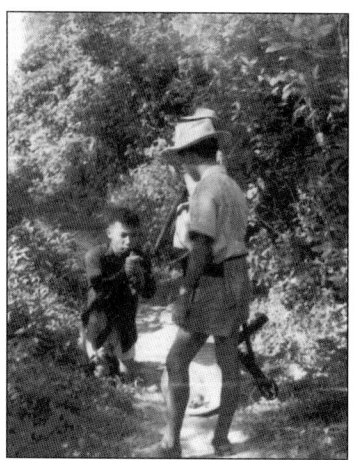
Viet Minh capture

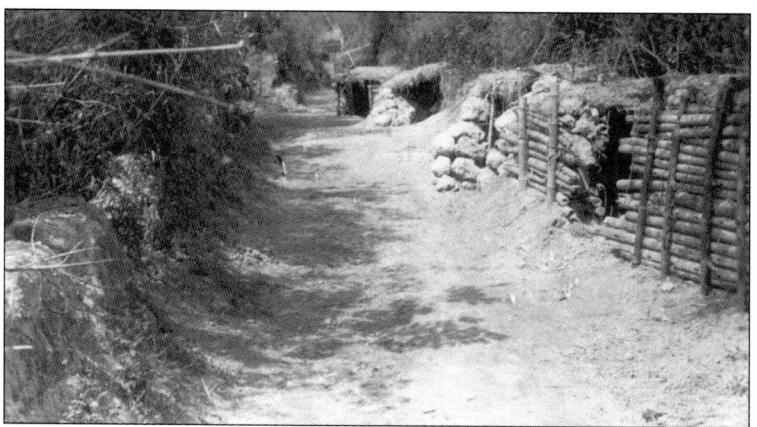
French forces — Nam Dinh

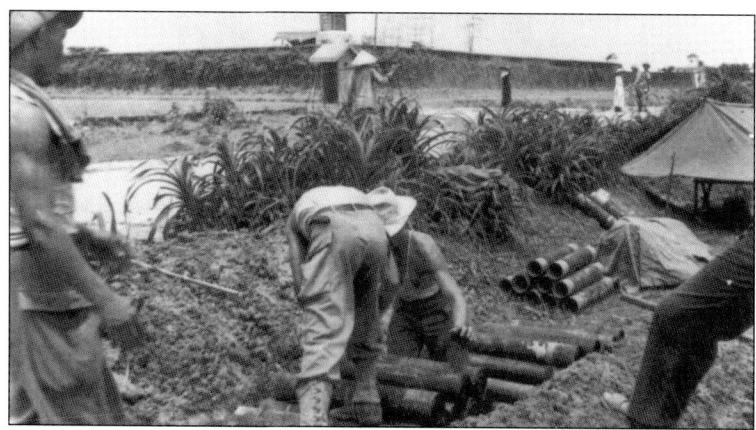
French forces — Nam Dinh

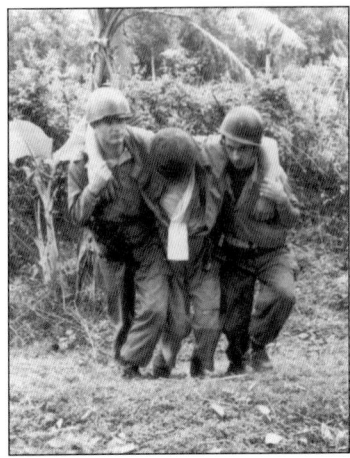
Wounded at Nam Dinh

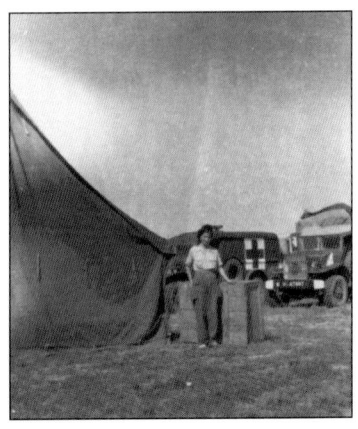
Elisabeth at medical tent — Nam Dinh

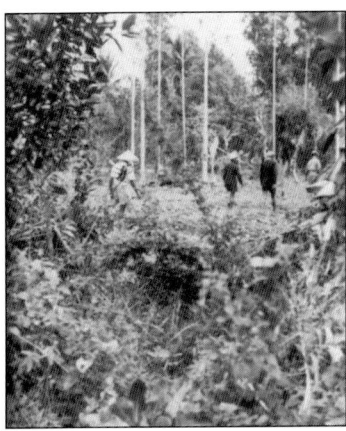
Nam Dinh

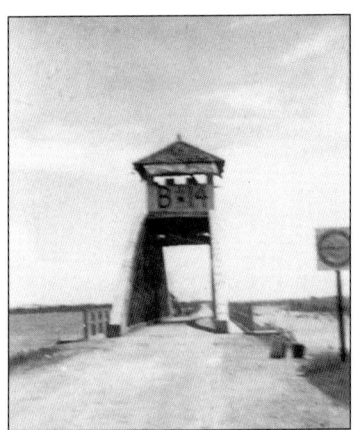
Lookout tower

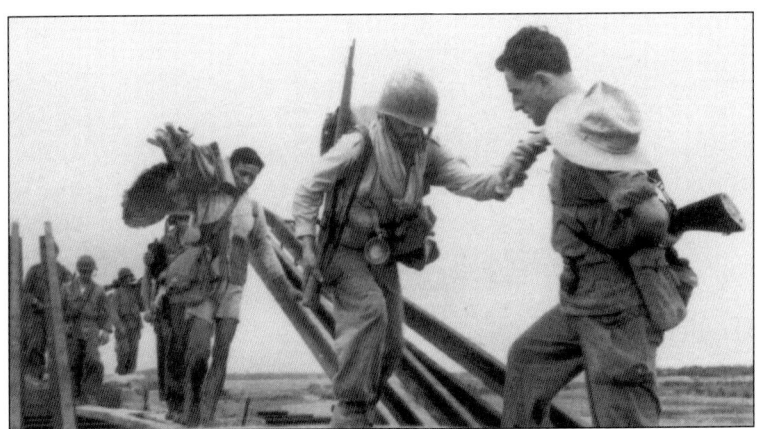
Troops crossing river near Nam Dinh

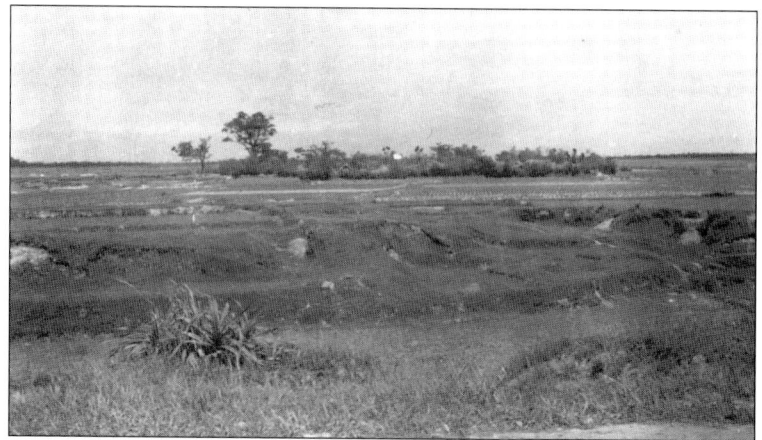
Going to Nam Dinh

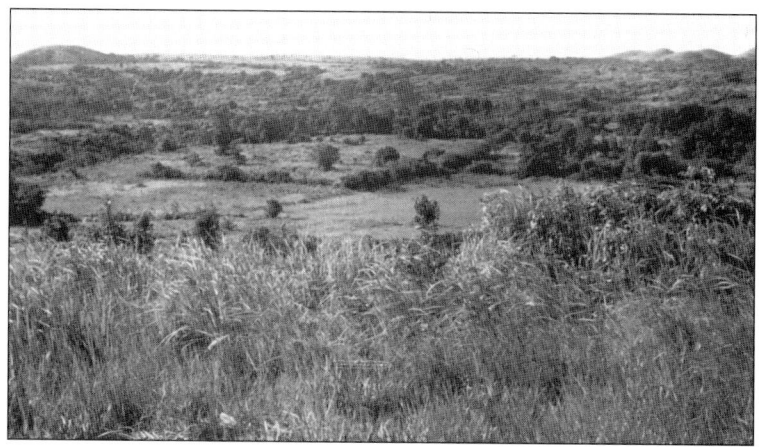
Going to Nam Dinh

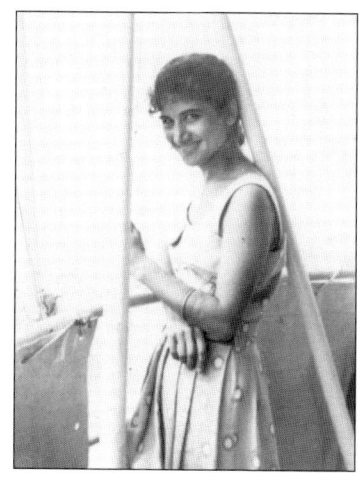
Elisabeth at 70 pounds

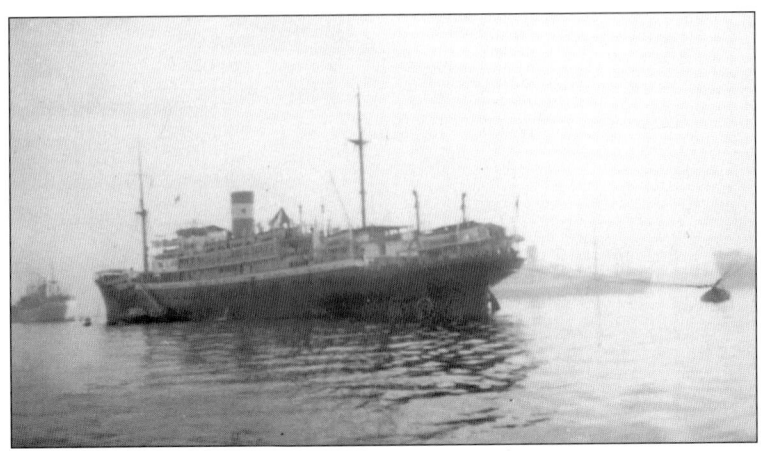

S.S. Kerquelen

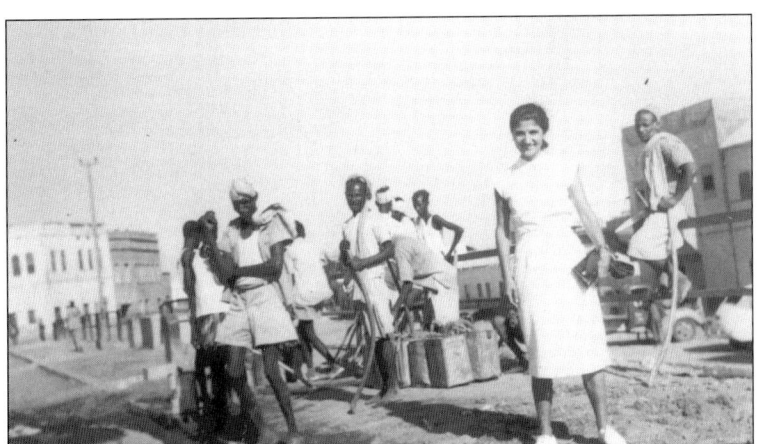

Colombo

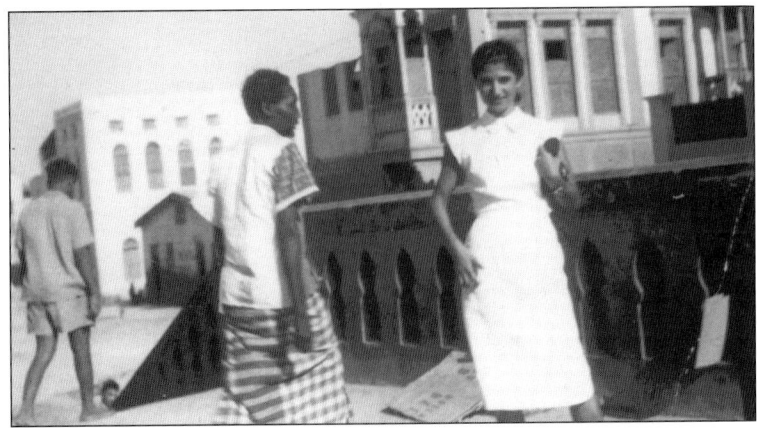

Singapore

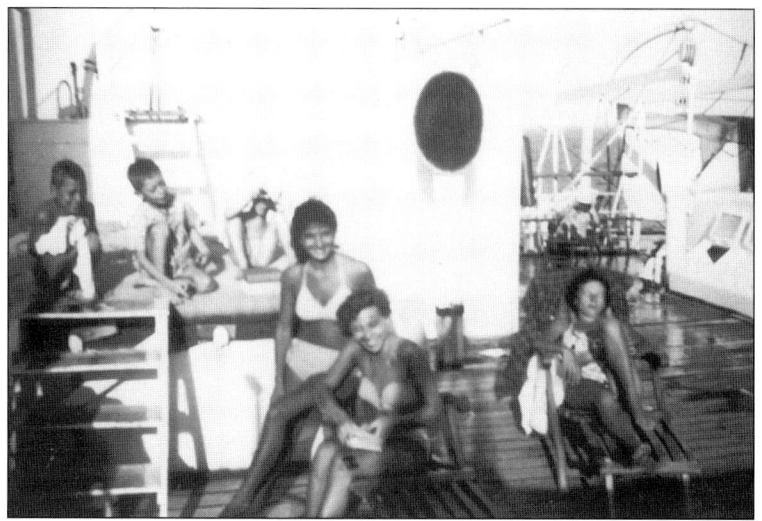

Nurses enjoying sun

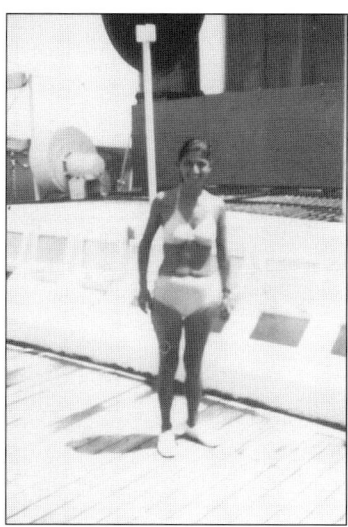

Elisabeth on deck

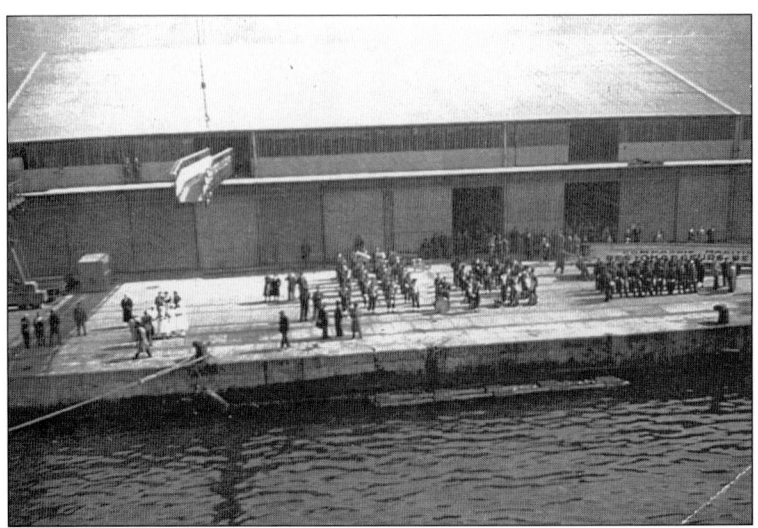

Homecoming ceremony — Marseilles

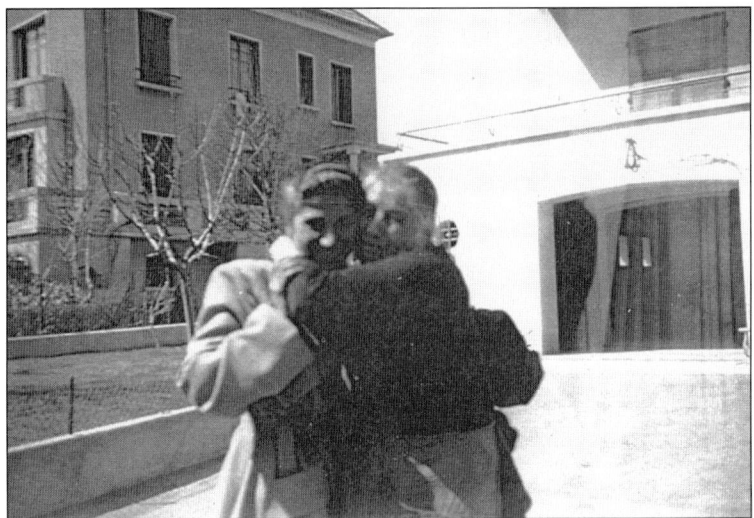

Elisabeth and Maman

Chapter 13
Home at Last

I took the train from Marseilles to Gap where Maman lived part of the year with my Aunt and Uncle Takvorian. Gap is located in the middle of the high Alps and only 150 kilometers from Marseilles. It is a beautiful city in a valley surrounded by high mountains. I arrived at noon and took a taxi to my relatives' home. I had not informed Maman I was coming home and had not called since arriving in France. As the taxi drove up to the house, I noticed Maman and Uncle Takvorian in the yard. Maman yelled, "It is Elisabeth," and came running to greet me. We hugged and kissed for a few minutes and Maman began to cry. I asked her why, and she said she always cried when she was so happy. I kissed Aunt Monique and Uncle Takvor and we went inside the house to talk. Uncle Takvor called all the rest of the family as soon as we were inside. Maman was still crying, almost in shock at my unexpected arrival. (Perhaps I should have called her from Marseilles, but I thought the suspense of waiting for me to get home would have been too much for her.) I spent the rest of the day bringing the family up to date on my experiences in Indochina. All my cousins who were living in Gap came over and we had a big party in the garden that evening. I went to bed early because I was emotionally tired and though I was back up to 80 pounds, I was still weak from my bout with typhoid and dysentery.

I spent most of my time with my cousin, Suzanne. She was 19 years old and had just finished high school. We became fast friends and visited many of the small towns near Gap. We also went to Grasse and visited a perfume factory where we both purchased some expensive fragrances. Suzanne was a beautiful girl and had been my playmate in Paris before World War II.

I reported to the Veterans Hospital in Paris (Val de Grace) on April 24, 1953. I met Angele and Sarah who were already there when I arrived. I was assigned to the hospital as a circulating nurse and Angele and Sarah were assigned as ward nurses. We lived in quarters at the hospital which had been a convent. It was constructed in 1645 and had been converted into a military hospital after the French Revolution. It was a beautiful place and we enjoyed working there. Most of our patients were from Indochina but there were also many disabled veterans from World War II still being treated. Many of the older veterans lived at the hospital.

We worked hard but thoroughly enjoyed our time off. Angele, Sarah, and I took every opportunity to reacquaint ourselves with Paris. We all loved to go to the movies and went at least once a week. I was eligible for discharge on July 18, 1953, and decided to leave the army and look for a job in Paris as a nurse. They held a big going-away party for me at the hospital and I was discharged the next day.

I took a small apartment in Paris and began searching for a position, but a surplus of nurses made a job very difficult to find. Fortunately, I had saved a lot of money while in Indochina and could afford to be off work for awhile. However, I became restless and contacted Margaret who lived in Verdun. She was happy to hear from me because her husband had just departed for duty in Indochina. She invited me to come and live with her on the family farm. She was the same Margaret I had known in Indochina and we both were happy to be together again.

She knew some people who were working at the large American Army base in Verdun so I applied there for work.

Within a week after my interview, I was assigned as the payroll clerk for French civilians working on the base. I bought a beautiful green Vespa, a small motorcycle, for $500.00 and I stayed with Margaret for three months. However, as winter approached, I moved into town to be closer to work; I did not wish to ride a long distance in the cold weather. I found a two-bedroom apartment with a small kitchen, a combined living and dining room, and one bathroom.

The American base had a movie theater and I was allowed to attend free. I utilized this opportunity to watch every film. I paid special attention to the language at work and in the theater and learned enough English to get by relatively well.

I called Maman and invited her to come and live with me in Verdun. She came two weeks later but with a surprise: Suzanne was with her. My sister was seven months pregnant and had left her legionnaire husband because of his abuse and heavy drinking. It was crowded but we got along very well. Suzanne delivered her baby boy, Jeannot, two months later. He was beautiful and healthful. I enjoyed having Maman and Suzanne with me, especially during the Christmas season. It was the first Christmas we had been together since 1949. Maman and Suzanne left Verdun and returned to Maman's Paris apartment in the middle of January 1954.

Margaret and I got together every weekend. Most of the time, I went to her farm and helped with the chores. In late January, Margaret learned that her husband died in Vietnam, where he was buried. Margaret was devastated, but I helped her through her grief. I spent most of my time at her home, staying overnight frequently. She was such a courageous woman, able to carry on and take care of her parents in spite of her anguish. Her depression was compounded because she had never had a child: "Part of him would still be alive if we had had children."

I enjoyed working with the Americans and corresponded frequently with the Carlsons who were still in Vietnam. I had made up my mind; I would go to America and attend a university. I began saving money and applying for various schools in the United States. After a year, a month before my 28th birthday, I left for the United States, where I have made a life and created a family of my own.

Epilogue

The French Indochina War effectively ended with the French defeat at Dien Bien Phu on the morning of May 8, 1954. France had suffered 32,800 casualties and an additional 12,000 Vietnamese soldiers loyal to France had been killed during the conflict. In addition, thousands of French soldiers were missing and never accounted for by either government. At the Geneva Conference of 1954, Vietnam was provisionally divided, pending nationwide free elections, into communist North Vietnam and nationalist South Vietnam. Fearing a communist victory, the regime of Ngo Dinh Diem refused to hold the scheduled elections and declared the south an independent republic in 1955. The Vietnam war ensued, with the United States aiding South Vietnam. I was unhappy with the defeat of our forces in Indochina and though I knew it was going to happen, I had not expected the end of French involvement so soon after I left the country.

I left Paris by air on November 5, 1955 and arrived in the United States that same day. At last, my longtime dream of visiting America was realized. I obtained a position as a nurse at a French Hospital in New York City where I worked for six months. Since I spoke Spanish more fluently than English, I moved to El Paso, Texas, to become a pediatric nurse at the Hotel Dieu Hospital and attended the University of Texas. I lived with a Mexican-American family near the hospital.

In February 1958, I met a young Army officer, Robert W. Sevier, and we dated from that time until we were married on July 24, 1958. I continued to attend the university part-time and worked at Hotel Dieu until Robert was reassigned to a missile site in Hecker, Illinois, in 1959.

We left El Paso and settled in the small town of Hecker (population 300) where I obtained a job at St. Clements Hospital in Red Bud as a circulating nurse in the operating room. I became a citizen of the United States in 1962. Still haunted by images of sick and wounded humans, especially children, I decided to quit nursing and become a teacher. In 1964, when Robert was serving an unaccompanied tour as a military advisor for the Republic of China in Taiwan, I enrolled at Belleville Community College in Belleville, Illinois. In 1968, we were transferred to White Sands Missile Range in New Mexico where Robert was assigned as a Missile Test Officer for the Safeguard System. I transferred to New Mexico State University in Las Cruces and graduated in May of 1971 with a B.S. degree in Education, majoring in French and Spanish.

I worked at Radford School for Girls in El Paso as a French and Spanish teacher from 1971 to 1975 when I resigned because we adopted a child from Mexico. I returned to work in 1977 in Sunland Park, New Mexico, and in 1978 I started work at the Gadsden School District near Ysleta, Texas, where I taught a Title-1 course for immigrant children.

Robert had retired from the United States Army in 1972, returned to school and obtained an accounting degree. In 1980, we moved to Oklahoma City where Robert took a position with the Federal Deposit Insurance Corporation as a bank examiner. In 1980, I obtained a position as a French and Spanish teacher at Edmond Memorial High School where I worked until I retired in May 1996.

Roger was killed in the Korean War. Dr. Carlson died in 1990 and Mrs. Carlson died in Colorado during 1995. In the mid-1990s, when I returned to France for a visit, I found out that Margaret had passed away also. Maman died in 1965 and Suzanne lives in the south of France.

Endnotes

1. During the summer of 1950, the Viet Minh infiltrated Saigon perpetuating terrorism and assassinations. The propaganda even affected school children who planned their own demonstrations. The police were powerless until a new prime minister and police chief were hired to rid the city of the communists. See Lucien Bodard, *The Quicksand War: Prelude to Vietnam* (Canada: Little, Brown & Company, 1967), 172–88.

2. Tons of ammunition, 13 howitzers, 940 machine guns, 450 vehicles, and 4,000 new submachine guns, 8,000 rifles, and thousands of gallons of gasoline were left behind at Lang Son alone. See Edgar O'Ballance, *The Indo-China War 1945–1954: A Study in Guerilla Warfare* (London: Faber & Faber, 1964), p. 118; The Committee of Concerned Asian Scholars, *The Indochina Story: A Fully Documented Account* (New York: Pantheon Books, 1970), p. 18; and Bernard Fall, *Two Vietnams: A Political and Military Analysis* (New York, 1967), p. 107.

3. After being run out of Saigon in 1950, the Viet Minh, led by Nguyen Binh, tried to capture the rich rice country around the city of Cantho. They planned a three-stage attack against regular French troops and were crushed by superior fire and air power. The Viet Minh never had a strong, concentrated force in South Vietnam again. Bodard, *The Quicksand War*, 196–98.

4. Of the 10,000 men posted at the northern border, 6,000 were killed during the 1950 Viet Minh offensive. Lt. Gen. Phillip B. Davidson, *Vietnam at War: The History 1946–1975* (Novato, CA: Presidio Press, 1988), p. 91; Ibid; Ibid.

5. *Fasciolopsis buski* is one of the most common species of trematode (parasite) in Asia. It is acquired by eating raw plants, such as water chestnuts. The patient can experience ulceration, hemorrhage, chronic diarrhea, and abscess of the intestinal wall. See L. Roberts and J. Janovy, Jr., *G.D. Schmidt and Larry S. Roberts' Foundations of Parasitology, 6th edition* (Boston: McGraw-Hill, 2000), pp. 259–60.

6. See Jacques Dalloz, *The War in Indochina, 1945–1954* (Savage, MD: Barnes and Noble, Ltd., 1990), pp. 138–39.

7. The alliance between France and the United States was complicated and duplicitous. The United States, initially critical of the Vichy government in Indochina had originally hoped that Chiang Kai-Shek would maintain his hold on China and eventually liberate Indochina from French colonialism. However, the United States was even more fearful of the Moscow-backed Chinese communists than the evils of colonialism and with Mao Tse-tung's victory over Kai-Shek in 1949, America was compelled to back the French to prevent the Indochinese dominoes from falling to the communists. The French, starved for domestic support, desperately needed American capital to hold onto their interests in the region. Thus, a strained alliance was created: French personnel held off the communists with American supplies and money, while American troops concentrated their anti-communist efforts in Korea. For a detailed account, see Bodard, *The Quicksand War*, pp. 220–30; also, Dalloz, *The War in Indochina*, pp. 143–45.

8. Though 700,000 troops were serving the French Army at the beginning of 1950, 54,000 Moroccans, Algerians, and Senegalese; 45,000 regular troops from Indochina; and 68,000 European troops, including legionnaires, made up the French Expeditionary Forces in the colony. Never more than 100,000 French, including civilians, were stationed by the army in Indochina at any time during the colonial war. Dalloz, *The War in Indochina*, p. 104.

9. In surveys taken between 1945–54, no more than 30% of the French population had any opinions about the conflict in Indochina. Dalloz, *The War in Indochina*, p. 103.

10. Though the Vichy government was allowed to operate in Indochina during World War II, in March of 1944, the Japanese set out to eliminate white domination in the land. Secret police terrorized and massacred the French colonists. After Japan surrendered to the Allies, Ho Chi Minh took advantage of the panicked French to fuel his people's revolution. His troops took over where the Japanese left off in torturing and killing the white population. Though British and French troops eventually drove the People's Republican Army back into the northern jungles, Vietnam would never revert to the passive colony it had been prior to World War II. Bodard, *The Quicksand War*, pp. 6–14.

11. The northeast (winter) monsoon, which generally affected the coast of central Vietnam from September through December, was not as severe as the southwestern monsoon. However, central Vietnam still received three downpours every day. The southwestern monsoon was most powerful in the south, but affected the whole country from May to October. For further description of the monsoons and how they affected military operations, see Davidson, *Vietnam at War*, p. 37 and throughout.

12. Religion played a major part in the war against the Viet Minh. The country was divided into countless religious sects, each with a particular agenda, and sometimes with fickle political loyalties. The Catholic minority was initially pro-nationalist after World War II. However, as Ho Chi Minh's policy of strict communism became more clear, Catholic sentiment changed. In addition, the French government solicited Pope Pius XII, a notorious anti-communist, for his blessing which they received, solidifying Vietnamese Catholics against the Viet Minh. See Dalloz, *The War in Indochina*, pp. 14–15, 111 and Bodard, *The Quicksand War*, pp. 29–33, 210–15.

13. Of the four different species of *Plasmodium* (parasite) that are carried by the *Anopheles* mosquito, *falciparum* is by far the most deadly. It often affects more peripheral blood cells than the chronic forms and can affect the brain, spleen, and bone marrow, where it can cause death. If left untreated, malignant malaria can cause massive lysis of blood cells, deadly blackwater fever. See Roberts and Janovy, Jr., *Foundations of Parasitology* (2000) which states that *falciparum* malaria accounts for 50% of all cases and is "the greatest killer of humanity in tropical zones," p. 1480.

14. The seafaring Cham people controlled central and southern Vietnam from approximately 100 A.D. through the 5th century. In 1217, the Khmers and Cham people united, but by the 17th century they lost their empire to the current Vietnamese people. For more information about this lost culture, see www.viettouch.com/vietnam_champa.html.

15. General Vo Nguyen Giap's rationale for moving operations in Laos included a plan to further erode French support for an ever-expanding war. He also knew that the French could not support their Laotian holdings without great effort and without depleting forces within the Tonkin area. For details about

General Vo Nguyen Giap's plan for Laos, see Davidson, *Vietnam at War*, pp. 148–53.

16. The Indochinese Federation was first announced on 1 November 1946 and established the following March. For details on the agreement signed by Ho Chi Minh, which reestablished Vietnam as a French colony, see Dalloz, *The War in Indochina*, p. 69.

17. At the beginning of 1952, the Viet Minh had as many as 125,000 regular troops, heavily supplied with Chinese machine guns and mortars. The Viet Minh expanded operations in central Vietnam and in January 1953 (6 months after Elisabeth noticed increased casualties in and around Hue) mounted major assaults on An Khe and Pleiku. The French managed to fend off the Viet Minh, but expeditionary forces were further spread out and drained. Davidson, *Vietnam at War*, pp. 137, 148.

18. The purpose of the 2,000-year-old pots remains a mystery. Legend says that they were giant vats for rice whiskey, but some scientists believe that they were funeral urns. About 350 stone pots can be seen at Thong Hai Hin, The Plain of Jars. See www.itisnet.com.

19. Chronic forms of malaria (*P. Ovale* and *P. Vivax*) can cause relapses throughout the lifetime of an infected person. While *falciparum* malaria does not relapse, patients can experience recrudescences up to three years after initial infection. Dr. Ralene Mitschler, Western Maryland College, personal correspondence, May 1999.

Additional Sources

For further comprehensive information, including detailed CIA maps, historical details and photographs, and cultural information about Vietnam and Laos, see www.christiantraveller.org and linked sites.

For modern color photographs of Vietnam, including the Perfume River, Imperial Palace, Da Lat and other sites Elisabeth mentions, see www.egr.msu.edu/~nguyenh4/two.html and www.metalab.unc.edu/vietnam.

For information on leprosy see www.who.int/lep.

For information on malaria, including latest statistics, see www.who.int/ctd/html/malaria.html

For information on other tropical diseases, including parasitic infections, see specific topics at the World Health Organization Web sites at www.who.org.

APPENDIX

OFFICIAL MILITARY RECORDS AND DOCUMENTS

ELISABETH KAPELIAN

MINISTÈRE
de la
DÉFENSE NATIONALE
(GUERRE)

CABINET

BUREAU
DES DÉCORATIONS

RÉPUBLIQUE FRANÇAISE

MÉDAILLE COLONIALE

Le Ministre

certifie que *L'A.T.A.T. de 5e Catégorie Kapelian Elisabeth* N° 387
du Détachement Autonome des Infirmiers C° des FFFS

Vu et enregistré au
Ministère de la Défense
Nationale (Guerre) sous le
304510

26 juillet 1893, avec agrafe: Extrême-Orient.

(Décret du 5 Août 1946)

A SAIGON, le 10 JUIL 1951 19___

Pour le Secrétaire d'État aux Forces
Armées et par Délégation
Pour le Général d'Armée de LATTRE de TASSIGNY
Haut-Commissaire de France en Indochine
et Commandant en Chef en Extrême-Orient
Le Général de Division SALAN
Adjoint Militaire

```
                                      I° REGION MILITAIRE
                                      ─────────────────
                                      COMPAGNIE D'ETAT-MAJOR
                                      DES TROUPES COLONIALES
                                      ─────────────────
                                      Caserne Clignancourt
                                            PARIS 18e
                                      Service : P.F.A.T.
```

CERTIFICAT DE LIBERATION DU SERVICE MILITAIRE

NOM __KAPELIAN__   Prénoms __Elizabeth__

Epouse _____

Née le __15-12-26__ à __Larissa (Grèce)__

Unité Numéro __CEMTC__   Spécialité __Infirmière__

Numéro Matricule __387/1921__   Catégorie __4ème__

Date de libération et motif __17-7-53 (fin de contrat)__

Adresse où se retire l'intéressée __Verdun - Meuse - 18 Rue de l'__
__7e Division Blindée USA__

Affectations successives __CEMTC - Extrême-Orient__
__CEMTC__

Signature de l'intéressée :
__J. Kapelian__

```
    Empreintes digitales
      des deux pouces
    [fingerprints]
```

PARIS, le __20 JUIL 1953__ 195
Le Capitaine BERTHON, Major de la
Compagnie d'Etat-Major des Troupes
                Coloniales,

[signature and stamp]

DESTINATAIRES :
- Intéressée
- Dossier de l'intéressée
- Recrutement et statistique I°R.M.
- Archives

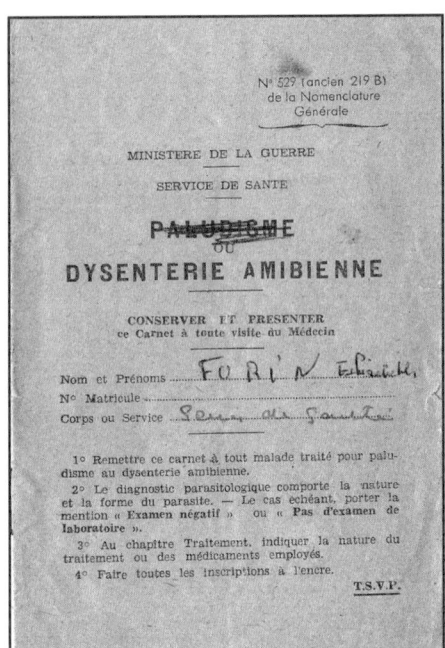

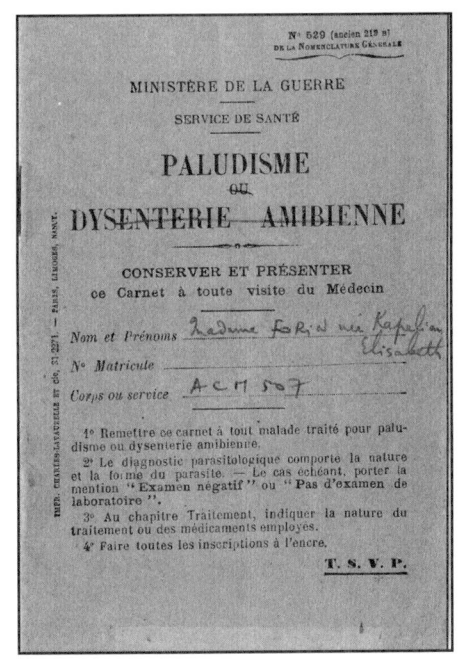

Name and first name: KAPELIAN, Elisabeth.   Serial Number: 45-758-08046.
(born the 12.15.1924 in Larissa (Greece))

DETAILS OF SERVICES AND TRANSFERS

Services and transfers	Date	References
Enlisted voluntarily for the duration of the war at the induction center of Belfort with the title of UA 8 the	2.21.45	Enlistment confirmed
Assigned to the infirmary AFAT the	2.21.45	9/ 1762
Transfered to the military Post Office.	2.21.45	AM n°5172 on the 9.24.45
Transfered to the 32nd UA in Paris with the intention of obtaining her discharge.		AM 5381 on the 2.1.46
Discharged by the 32nd UA the	3.7.46	Slip n°754
Reenlisted for two years at the induction center of Paris with the title of C.E.F.E.O. the	3.24.50	Enlistment confirmed S/n°119
Assigned to the C.R.P.F.I. of Margival the	3.24.50	
Transfered to the military hospital D.Larrey in Versailles.	3.24.50	
Classified 5th category alc	3.24.50	D.7894/RA
Assigned to the S.I.C.I. Indochina with the title of nurse's aid.	6.11.50	AM 1520
Left Paris the	8.17.50	8112.50
Landed in Saigon the	8.20.50	
Was appointed to the service of Dr. Colonel DGS TFUS hlc	8.22.50	AM 6996/ DSS/1
Assigned DAIC/FFVS, chief of Saint Jacques		AM 2149
Promoted 5th category 2nd Grade alc	12.15.50	8.24.50
Promoted 5th category 3rd Grade hlc	6.15.51	D.79 5.25.50
Assigned to the DAIC/TCV at the service of the Dr. Colonel, director of health services of the land forces of the Vietman Center.		AM 8523 DSS 7.10.51
Arrived at the unit and admitted there	7.20.51	
Assigned A.C.M. 507		AM 2989. 7.20.50
Assigned to the infirmary of the garrison of Tourane		AM 1543/SCA 4.8.52
Given permission to stay two more years in Indochina		D.1887/DSS 4.30.52
Promoted to the 4th category alc	1.1.52	D.886- 5.9.52
Reenlisted for six months with the title of DAIC/CV at the military post of Tourane.	3.24.52	Enlistment confirmed S/ 525
Given permission to extend her stay in EO for six months alc	8.20.52	D.22281 7.13.52

Subscribed before me this 10th day of February, 1965.

Transcribed and certified conforme to the original

Christiane M. Ahorn

SERVICE RECORDS (CONTINUED)

1st Region	Department: Seine
Name: KAPELIAN First Name: Elisabeth Divorced: Forin Married Name: SEVIER,	Serial Number: 45-758-08046

DETAILS OF SERVICES AND TRANSFERS: (Continued)

Services and Tranfers	Date	References
Reenlisted for six months with the title of DALC/CV at the hlc military Post of Tourane as a nurse	9.24.52	Enlistment paper S/n° 740 Am 239/DSS
Transfered to the SICX Indochina (RPA)	1.10.53	on the 2.13.53.
Repatriated for the rest of the duration of the enlistment		
Embarked on the S.S. KERGUELEN the	2.25.53	
Landed in Marseille the	3.23.53	
On furlough from the 3.24 to the	7.17.53	
Attached to the C.E.M.T.C. hlc	2.25.53	
Discharged the	7.18.53	as a nurse.

* Declared her intention to live
 in Verdun, 15 rue de la Division
 Blindee USA also serve as a agent P1   *1 has served.
 from the 5.1.1944 to the 9.30.1944.
 in the network of Jean Marie Buckmaster
 of the French fighting forces.
 (Attestation FFC n° 59,971 on the 1.27.49.

Certified conforme to the
original.
Commandant of the Recruiting Center.
26 August 1961.

Subscribed before me this 19th day of February, 1965.

signature
Notary Public
My Commission Expires November 7, 1968

Translated and certified conforme to the original
Christiane Shoop

SERVICE RECORDS (CONTINUED)

```
Name: KAPELI..                          Serial Number:
First Name: Elisabeth                   45-758-08046
Divorced: Perin
Married Name: SEVIER
```

Campaigns			Citations and Rewards	Decorations
from the	to the	against		
5.1.44	9.30.44	US ???	Cited to the order of the ?????? (n°783) on the 4.??.??: "Young nurse with remarkable courage, served from May 19?? until the liberation, the cause of the resistance with an abnegation worthy of praise. Was a nurse in the Maquis of Etang Neuf (Yonne). Devoted herself to the care of the wounded and sick" A	Commemorative Medal 39-45 pin EV Bronze Croix de Guerre. Colonial Medal, pin EO (Patent n°304510) on the 7.10.51. Commemorative Medal of the campaign of Indochina.
2.21.45	1.8.45	CD army		
8.17.50	8.20.50	1/2 a Air		
8.21.50	2.24.53	CD EO		
2.25.53	3.23.53	1/2 a sea		
3.24.53	7.17.53	CD CFC		
			Has always shown even in the most dangerous conditions, outstanding courage. This citation includes the Croix de Guerre in bronze.	

Translated conformed to the original
Christiane M Ahoop

Subscribed before me this 10th day of February, 1965

Notary Public
My Commission Expires November 7, 1966

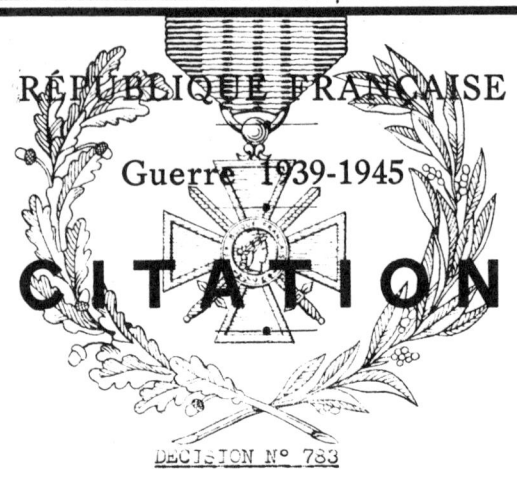

RÉPUBLIQUE FRANÇAISE

Guerre 1939-1945

CITATION

DECISION N° 783

LE SECRETAIRE D ETAT AUX FORCES ARMEES " GUERRE "

CITE   A L ORDRE DU REGIMENT

KAPELIAN Elisabeth   -   (F.F.C.)

" Jeune infirmière, ayant un courage remarquable, a servi la cause de la résistance avec une abnégation digne d'éloges. De Mai 1944 à la libération, infirmière du maquis dans l'Yonne, a prodigué ses soins aux blessés et aux malades. A toujours montré même dans les circonstances les plus critiques un dévouement et un mépris du danger hors de pair."-

CETTE CITATION COMPORTE L ATTRIBUTION DE LA CROIX DE GUERRE AVEC ETOILE DE BRONZE, ET ELLE ANNULE ET REMPLACE CELLES ACCORDEES ANTERIEUREMENT POUR LES MEMES FAITS.-

FAIT à PARIS, le 15 Juin 1948

Signé : Max LEJEUNE

POUR AMPLIATION
PARIS, le 15 Juin 1948
L Administrateur de 1° Cl.
BAUMONT
Chef du Bureau Décorations
P/O. Le Capitaine LAMOTHE

THE FRENCH REPUBLIC

WORLD WAR II 1939-1943
CITATION # 783

The Secretary of the Armed Forces granted by the order of the Regiment to

Kapelian, Elisabeth
F.F.C.
Combatant in the French Forces

A young nurse, displaying remarkable courage, has served the cause of the Resistance with praiseworthy self-sacrifice from May 1944 to the liberation, as a nurse in the Resistance in the Department of Yonne. She has prodigiously tended for the sick and the wounded, always demonstrating even in the most critical circumstances a dedication to duty and a disdain for danger beyond compare.

This honor includes the granting of the Cross of War with Bronze Star and it supersedes all other awards previously granted for the same accomplishments.

Traduit par
Phyllis Laws
30-4-43

Subscribed and sworn to before me this _3_ day of _May_ 19_93_.
My commission expires _4-15-97_.

Kathryn L. Anderson Notary Public

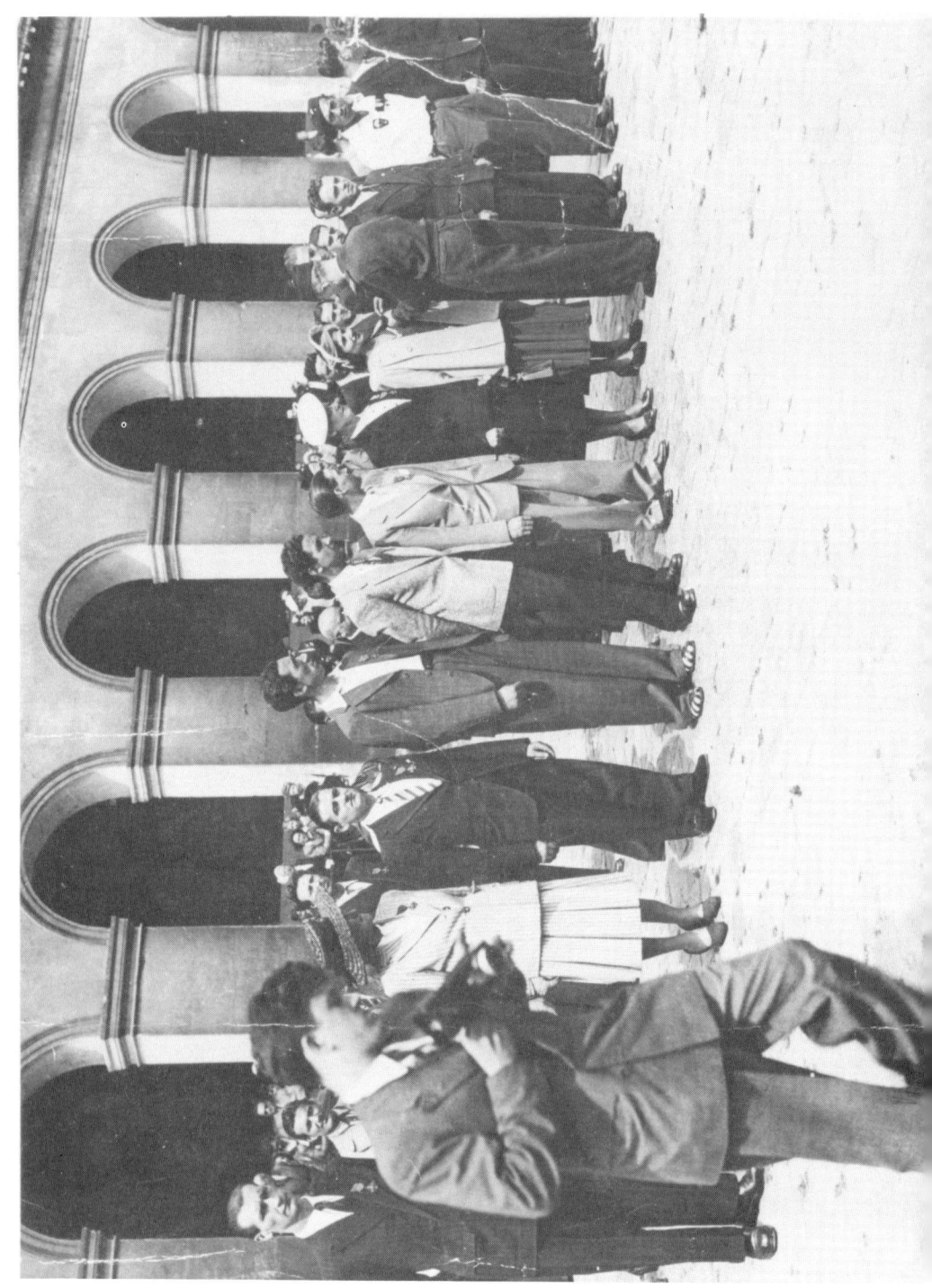
Ceremony where Elisabeth received Croix de Guerre for WWII service

OKLAHOMA 73013 U.S.A

PRÉFECTURE
DE PARIS
SERVICE DÉPARTEMENTAL
DE L' O.N.A.C.V.G.

RÉPUBLIQUE FRANÇAISE

MINISTÈRE
DES A[illegible]S COMBATTANTS
[illegible]MES DE GUERRE

CARTE DU C[illegible]TTANT

DÉLIVRÉE
EN APPLICATION DE LA DÉCISION [illegible] 49 300
N° 270790 [illegible] 1996

à Madame KAPELIAN/[illegible]
Prénoms Elisabeth
Domicile 2704 Blue Quail Pass Edmond
Né(e) le 15 12 1926, à LARISSA/ GRECE
A PARIS, le 13 JUIN 1996

LE TITULAIRE

LE SECRÉTAIRE GÉNÉRAL DU SERVICE DÉPARTEMENTAL
M. LARIVIÈRE

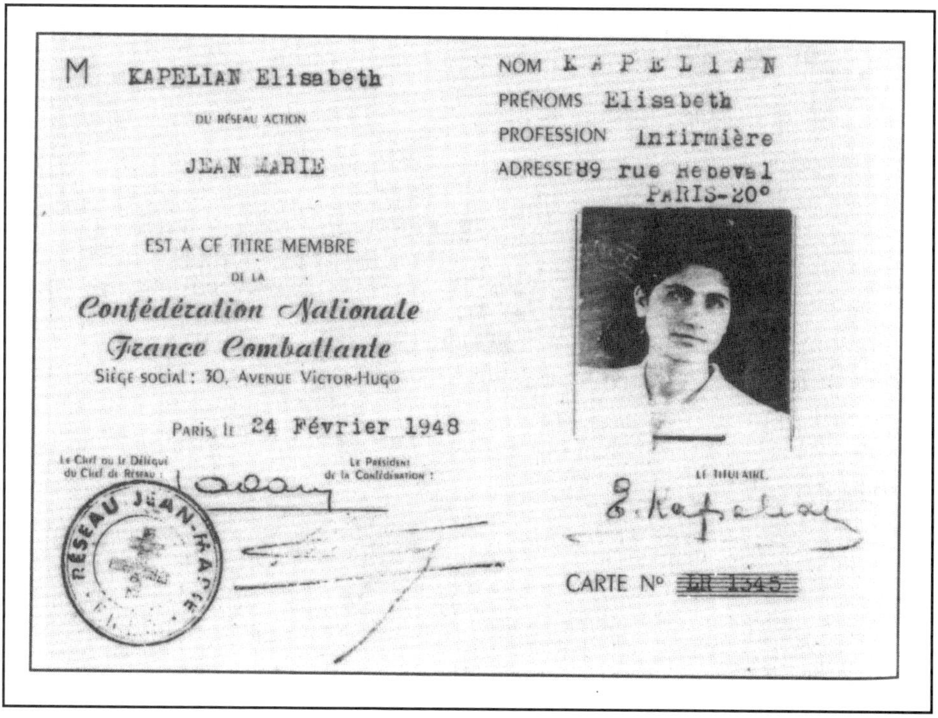

M KAPELIAN Elisabeth
DU RÉSEAU ACTION
JEAN MARIE
EST A CE TITRE MEMBRE
DE LA
Confédération Nationale
France Combattante
SIÈGE SOCIAL : 30, AVENUE VICTOR-HUGO
PARIS, LE 24 Février 1948

Le Chef ou le Délégué du Chef de Réseau :

Le Président de la Confédération :

RÉSEAU JEAN-MARIE

NOM KAPELIAN
PRÉNOMS Elisabeth
PROFESSION Infirmière
ADRESSE 89 rue Rebeval
PARIS-20°

LE TITULAIRE
E. Kapelian

CARTE N° LR 1345

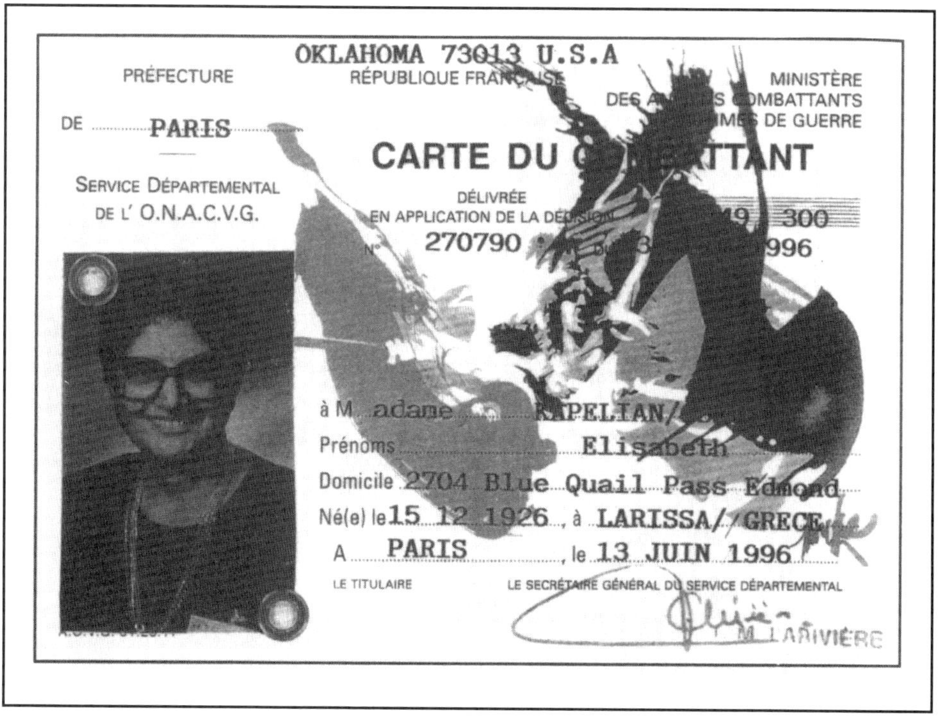

LE GÉNÉRAL DE GAULLE   COLOMBEY--LES-DEUX-EGLISES, le 20 JUILLET 1946

Mademoiselle,

    J'ai pris connaissance avec attention de la lettre que vous m'avez adressée.

    Vous ne manquerez pas d'être tenue informée de la suite qui aura pu être réservée à votre requête.

    Veuillez agréer, Mademoiselle, l'assurance de mes sentiments respectueux.

[signature]

Mademoiselle Lisette KAPELIAN
Salon Richard Wallace
Hopital Tenon
PARIS (20 ème)

General De Gaulle   COLOMBEY-LES-DEUX-EGLISES, 20 JULY 1945

Madmoiselle,

I have carefully considered the letter which you sent me.

I shall not fail to keep you informed of the outcome of the request which you sent me.

Please accept, Mademoiselle, my most respectful sentiments.

Signature

Mademoiselle Lisette KAPELIAN
Salon Richard Wallace
Hospital Tenon
Paris (20 eme)

Translated by: Phyllis Laws
Phyllis Laws

Subscribed and sworn to before me this 22 day of Sept 1993.
My commission expires April 15, 1997.

Kathryn R Anderson Notary Public

Other Books about the Life of Elisabeth Sevier

Resistance Fighter, A Teenage Girl in World War II France, E. Sevier, Sunflower University Press, 1537 Yuma, PO Box 1009, Manhattan, KS 66505-1009, Price $18.95. Order by telephone: 800-258-1232 or from your local bookseller.

Wesley Publishing Co.
2704 Blue Quail Pass
Edmond, OK 73013-8844
Telephone: 405-340-3436

To order copies of *War Without a Front*, please remit $18.95 check or money order for each copy. We will send by priority mail the day after receipt and pay the postage.

Discount offered for orders of 5 books or more. Please call for rate.

Please call for rates to booksellers.